The Physics of Clinical MR Taught Through Images

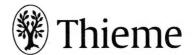

The Physics of Clinical MR Taught Through Images

Val M. Runge, M.D.
Robert and Alma Moreton Centennial Chair in Radiology
Department of Radiology, Scott and White Clinic and Hospital
Texas A&M University Health Science Center, Temple, Texas

Wolfgang R. Nitz, Ph.D.
Application Development
MR Division, Siemens Medical Solutions, Inc.
Erlangen, Germany;
Department of Radiology
University Hospital of Regensburg, Regensburg, Germany

Stuart H. Schmeets, B.S., R.T.(R)(MR)
Advanced Specialist, MRI Applications
Siemens Medical Solutions USA, Inc.
Malvern, Pennsylvania

William H. Faulkner, Jr., B.S., R.T.(R)(MR)(CT)
William Faulkner & Associates, L.L.C.
Director of Education, Chattanooga Imaging
Chattanooga, Tennessee

Nilesh K. Desai, M.D.
Department of Radiology
Parkland Health and Hospital System
The University of Texas Southwestern Medical Center
Dallas, Texas

Thieme Medical Publishers
New York • Stuttgart

Thieme New York
333 Seventh Avenue
New York, NY 10001

Senior Editor: Timothy Y. Hiscock
Assistant Editor: Birgitta Brandenburg
Director, Production and Manufacturing: Anne Vinnicombe
Senior Production Editor: David R. Stewart
Marketing Director: Phyllis Gold
Director of Sales: Ross Lumpkin
Chief Financial Officer: Peter van Woerden
President: Brian D. Scanlan
Compositor: Thomson Press (India) Limited
Printer: The Maple-Vail Book Manufacturing Group

Library of Congress Cataloging in Publication Data is available from the publisher

Important note: Medical knowledge is ever-changing. As new research and clinical experience broaden our knowledge, changes in treatment and drug therapy may be required. The authors and editors of the material herein have consulted sources believed to be reliable in their efforts to provide information that is complete and in accord with the standards accepted at the time of publication. However, in view of the possibility of human error by the authors, editors, or publisher of the work herein, or changes in medical knowledge, neither the authors, editors, or publisher, nor any other party who has been involved in the preparation of this work, warrants that the information contained herein is in every respect accurate or complete, and they are not responsible for any errors or omissions or for the results obtained from use of such information. Readers are encouraged to confirm the information contained herein with other sources. For example, readers are advised to check the product information sheet included in the package of each drug they plan to administer to be certain that the information contained in this publication is accurate and that changes have not been made in the recommended dose or in the contraindications for administration. This recommendation is of particular importance in connection with new or infrequently used drugs.

Some of the product names, patents, and registered designs referred to in this book are in fact registered trademarks or proprietary names even though specific reference to this fact is not always made in the text. Therefore, the appearance of a name without designation as proprietary is not to be construed as a representation by the publisher that it is in the public domain.

Printed in the United States of America

5 4 3 2

TNY ISBN 1-58890-322-2
GTV ISBN 3-13-140611-9

To my two daughters, Valerie and Sadie, with all my love

With special thanks to John E. Kirsch, Ph.D., for his technical expertise and review of the material included for accuracy, to Jilene Gendron, R.T., for her assistance in image acquisition, and to Wendy Amaral for her medical illustrations.

I would also like to express my sincere appreciation to the many members of the Radiology department at Scott and White, who by their hard work and support, both directly and indirectly, made this project possible.

Contents

Foreword

Magnetic resonance imaging (MRI) has proven itself to be the premiere imaging technique of the last two decades. Its soft tissue contrast exceeds that of computed tomography (CT) and ultrasound, based largely on the many tissue parameters that can be brought out by a well-designed pulsing sequence. These include not only the well-known fundamental parameters such as T1, T2, and proton density but also diffusion, chemical shift, susceptibility, and flow effects.

MRI physics has traditionally been taught through mathematical models such as the Bloch equation. While having a fundamental understanding of MRI at the mathematical level certainly offers considerable insight into MRI processes, most radiologists and physicians who rely on MRI do not have the mathematical sophistication to understand MRI in this manner. Most of us understand MRI through the effect of changing sequence parameters on image contrast.

Dr. Runge has done an excellent job of teaching "how MRI works" using MR images. His approach is very intuitive and easily grasped by those without a particularly strong mathematical background. Considering the complexity of the MR process, he should be lauded for conceiving and carrying out this simplifying approach.

This text should be useful for all radiologists who read MR studies, even on an occasional basis. In fact such radiologists are likely to benefit the most from this book as their understanding of MRI and their confidence in MR-based diagnosis increases.

It is an ideal text for medical students who are frequently baffled by the complex physics of MRI, often to the point of avoiding radiology altogether and going into other specialties such as surgery or internal medicine. This is a perfect text for radiology residents when they are first exposed to MRI. This book will help them gain from their early clinical experience as they acquire additional depth of understanding from the more traditional physics approach. Finally, this book is also ideal for nonradiologists who want to increase their working knowledge of MRI without spending a lot of time studying the physics.

I congratulate Dr. Runge on this book, which clearly fills a large void in the MR educational literature.

William G. Bradley, Jr., M.D., Ph.D., FACR
University of California, San Diego
San Diego, California

Preface

The objective of this textbook is to teach through images a practical approach to magnetic resonance (MR) physics and image quality. Unlike prior texts covering this topic, the focus is on clinical images rather than equations. A practical approach to MR physics is developed through images, emphasizing knowledge of fundamentals important to achieve high image quality. Pulse diagrams are also included, which many at first find difficult to understand. Readers are encouraged to glance at these as they go through the text. With time and repetition, as a reader progresses through the book, the value of these and the knowledge thus available will become evident (and the diagrams themselves easier to understand).

The text is organized into concise chapters, each discussing an important point relevant to clinical MR and illustrated with images from routine patient exams. The topics covered encompass the breadth of the field, from imaging basics and pulse sequences to advanced topics including contrast enhanced MR angiography, spectroscopy, perfusion, and diffusion. Discussion of the latest hardware and software innovations, for example multichannel phased array coil technology and parallel imaging, is included because these topics are critical to current and future advances.

The clinical applications and complexity of MR continue to increase. Progress in MR has largely dominated the field of diagnostic radiology for the past 20 years. Today MR stands as a major diagnostic subspecialty. The sophistication of this technique and continued advances dictate that MR will continue to play a dominant role in clinical medicine for the foreseeable future.

Val M. Runge, M.D.

The Physics of Clinical MR
Taught Through Images

1 Components of an MR Scanner: MR Basics in a Nutshell

◆ The Magnet

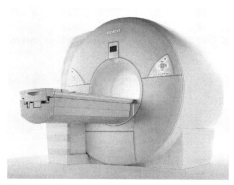

Figure 1–1

Hydrogen atoms have a nuclear spin, and associated with the nuclear spin is a magnetic moment. A strong magnetic field causes an orientation of those magnetic moments parallel to the magnetic field. The magnetic field strength B_0 is measured in tesla (T). A 1.5-T system (Fig. **1–1**) provides a magnetic field of about 30,000 times the earth's field, with no permanent effects on human physiology and negligible temporary alterations. The magnetic field is generated by feeding ~400 ampere (A) into superconductive windings. Superconductivity means that once the current flows, the power supply can be disconnected, the end and beginning of the coil windings connected, and the current will continue to flow. The magnet will be at field at all times, even during a power outage.

◆ The Transmitting Radiofrequency Coil

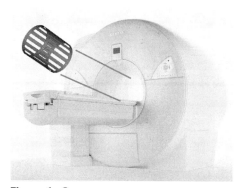

Figure 1–2

Tilting the magnetic moments away from the parallel orientation causes them to precess (spin with a motion in which their axis sweeps out a cone), with a Larmor frequency of ~42 MHz/T. These rotating magnetic moments induce an electromagnetic signal in adjacent coils—the so-called magnetic resonance (MR) signal. To tilt the magnetic moments, a rotating B_1 field is required that is rotating with the same frequency as the magnetic moments. Only those "in resonance" will be affected, hence the term *magnetic resonance*. An antenna transmitting a radiofrequency (RF) field provides the rotating B_1 field (Fig. **1–2**). A 90° RF excitation pulse with a duration of, for example, 2.5 ms provides a B_1 field of ~2.3 μT. The RF frequencies used are below that of microwaves, yet there may be some warming of the patient. The energy transferred is referred to as specific absorption rate (SAR), which, in normal mode, is up to 1.5 W/kg.

◆ The Gradients

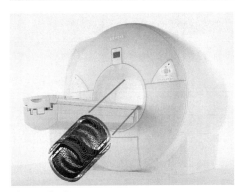

Figure 1 – 3

Currents driven through a gradient coil provide a smooth change in magnetic field strength along one direction, causing the magnetic moments to have different precessional frequencies depending on location.

The RF pulse can consist of a composition of frequencies, and only those magnetic moments in resonance with these frequencies will be excited— the basic principle of slice-selective excitation.

Once the magnetic moments rotate, magnetic field gradients can again be established to "encode" spatial information into the signal via the precessional frequencies. Magnetic field gradients are established by sending ~400 A through the resistive windings of a gradient coil (Fig. **1 – 3**) for 7 ms, for example, causing a field variation of 40 mT/m. The slew rate, reported in T/m/s is a measure of how fast the gradient can be established. All applications benefit from a fast and strong gradient system. Mechanical forces based on electromagnetic interactions between the windings of the gradient coil cause minor distortions in their shape, resulting in a knocking noise during the exam. Technology is advanced to the point where the patient is the limiting factor. Fast-changing magnetic field gradients induce currents in the patient's body (which is a poor conductor) and may mimic nerve signals causing unintended muscle contractions. A "stimulation monitor" assesses the setup and prevents execution of such protocols.

◆ The Receiver Coils

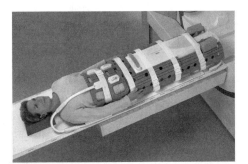

Figure 1 – 4

The main source for image noise in MR is the patient. The smaller the receiving coil (Fig. **1 – 4**), the less noise is picked up. The closer the coil is to the source of the MR signal, the greater the induced signal.

2 MR Safety: Static Magnetic Field

Magnetic resonance imaging (MRI) has become a mainstay of diagnostic imaging. When properly utilized it is very safe and effective. It remains, however, the only imaging modality in which a patient injury or death can occur almost instantly. Safety concerns exist with each type of magnetic field associated with an MR system: the static field (B_0), the radiofrequency field (B_1), and the gradient magnetic fields used for spatial encoding. In this case we focus on issues relating to the static magnetic field (B_0).

There are two types of forces exerted on a ferrous object when brought in close proximity to an MR magnet: translational and rotational. The rotational force is that which causes a ferrous object to turn and align with the direction of the magnetic field. Rotational forces are strongest at the isocenter of the magnet. Translational forces are those that cause a ferrous object to be pulled toward the magnet isocenter. Translational forces are actually near zero at the isocenter, because translational forces are felt when a ferrous object is in a magnetic field that changes in strength over distance. MRI requires a homogeneous magnetic field, and thus within the bore of a magnet the magnetic field usually changes very little. However, as one approaches an MR system, entering from the door of the scanner, the field strength begins to increase. The closer one gets to the magnet, the more severe the magnetic field changes. The more severe the change in the magnetic field, the greater the attractive force on a ferrous object. Most horizontal field (cylindrical) MR systems today are magnetically shielded to bring this fringe field closer to the magnet for siting purposes. As a result, the magnetic field changes very rapidly as one gets close to the magnet. Bringing a ferrous object into the room is extremely dangerous and should not be done. Many times, once one feels the pull of the magnetic field, it is too late. Fig. **2–1** shows the result of a floor buffer that was inadvertently brought into an MR scan room. There have been cases of injury and even a patient death resulting from ferrous oxygen tanks being brought into the scan room.

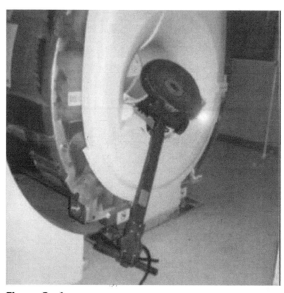

Figure 2–1

Vertical field (i.e., low field or so-called open MR) systems are not safer with regard to translational forces. Even though the magnetic field at the isocenter may be lower than the field strength of horizontal field (cylindrical) magnets, the change in the fringe field is actually quite severe near the magnet poles, going from near zero to the maximum in just a meter or two. The same precautions that one follows for high-field (1.5 T) cylindrical systems should be followed regardless of the MR system field strength or orientation. Additionally, for MR systems utilizing a permanent magnet design, one should remember that the magnet field cannot be "turned off" by any means. For all types of MR systems, access by non-MR personnel should be restricted, and warning signs, stating that the magnet is always on, are advocated.

The presence of implants and magnetically and/or electrically activated devices can pose serious hazards for anyone with such an implant or device entering the scan room. Anyone entering the scan room (or beyond the 5-gauss line) should be screened by trained MR personnel. This includes not only the patient but also any family members or support personnel. Most orthopedic implants, fortunately, are made from nonferromagnetic materials and are thus safe for MR.

If a the patient has some type of implant or device, it should be positively identified so that the physician in charge can determine if it is MR safe or if there is a significant risk such that the patient should be excluded from entering the MR scan room. It is the ultimate responsibility of the MR radiologist/physician to determine if a patient can safely undergo an MR procedure. With the advent of higher field MR systems (3.0 T or greater) it is important to remember that implants and/or devices that have been found safe at 1.5 T are not necessarily safe for imaging at 3.0 T. Up-to-date information about implant safety and testing can be found at *www.MRISafety.com.*

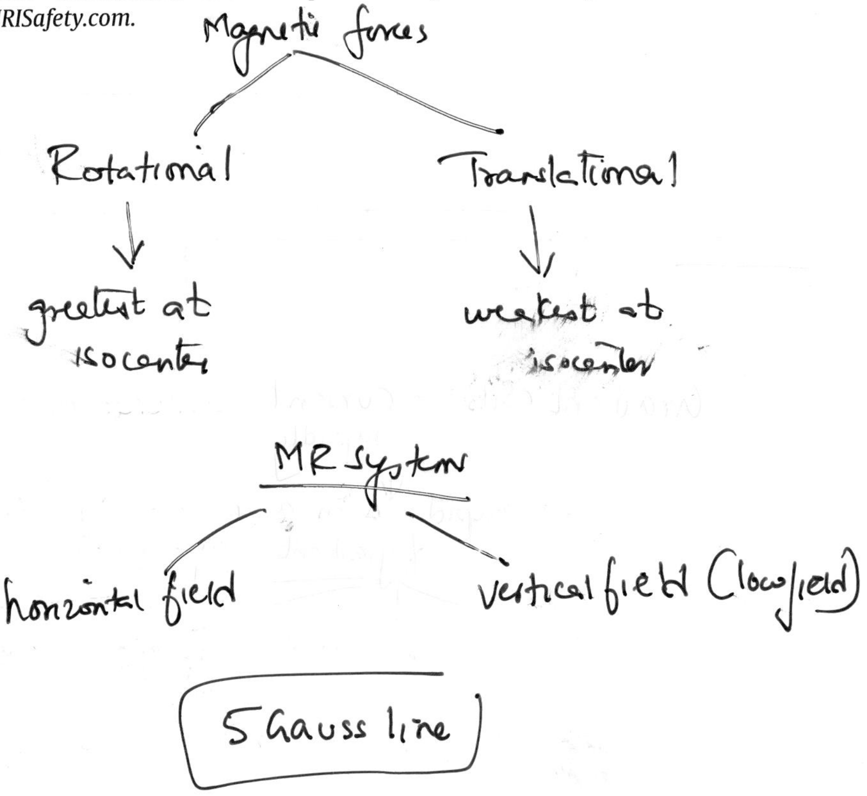

Handwritten annotations:

Magnetic forces
- Rotational → greatest at isocenter
- Translational → weakest at isocenter

MR System
- horizontal field
- vertical field (low field)

5 Gauss line

3 MR Safety: Gradient Magnetic Field

Gradient magnetic fields are used primarily for spatial encoding (localization) of the MR signal. Additional coils of wire located within the magnet bore (but underneath the plastic housing, and thus not visible to the patient or technologist) produce these fields. During scan acquisition, the current in the gradient coils is switched on and off rapidly, causing in turn quick changes in amplitude and polarity of the gradient magnetic fields. There are four primary performance-related characteristics that define a gradient system. These are slew rate (how fast one can drive a gradient to a specific amplitude), maximum amplitude (how high a gradient field one can actually achieve, regardless of how long it takes), spatial linearity (how far away from isocenter the gradient field reaches before its strength begins to fall off), and duty cycle (how often one can drive the gradient without failure). All four are very relevant to clinical performance. High slew rates permit shorter echo times (TEs) and echo spacing, improving the image quality of fast spin echo scans and contrast-enhanced MR angiography. High-amplitude gradients markedly improve diffusion weighted scans. Cost issues aside, there are constraints imposed upon gradient amplitude, slew rate, and spatial linearity due to nerve stimulation (which occurs above a certain dB/dt limit).

One very noticeable result from the rapid switching of the gradient coils is the acoustic noise. Pulsing the gradients creates a force (due to the magnetic field created around the wires) that generates pressure waves and thus the audible sound (knocking). Generally speaking, the higher the B_0, the higher the gradient field amplitude, and the faster the switching speed, the louder the acoustic noise. Many strategies have been used to reduce the sound to acceptable limits, and these continue to be developed. In many high-field MR systems, hearing protection of some type is necessary for patients and anyone in the scan room.

High dB/dt (rapid changes in the magnetic field) can also induce current in conductive leads and materials. There are documented incidents of current induction in surface coil wires, electrocardiogram (ECG) leads, and even implant leads leading to patient burns. Care should always be taken to position any wires or leads required for the MR study so that they do not form loops. Wires also should not be positioned so that they touch the patient directly, because a conductive loop can be formed between the wire and the patient.

Gradient coils — current switched on & off rapidly

rapid Δ in amplitude & polarity of gradient mag. fields

slew rate   max. amplitude   spatial linearity   duty cycle

4 MR Safety: Radiofrequency Magnetic Field

B_1

The radiofrequency (RF) field used in MRI is also referred to as the B_1 field. Its purpose is to excite the spins, creating an MR signal that can be detected by a receiver coil. The frequency at which the MR phenomenon can be induced is termed the Larmor frequency (f_0), which for protons (hydrogen nuclei) is 42.6 MHz/T. At 1.5 T, the f_0 is 63 MHz. The amount of RF power necessary for imaging is dependent on several factors. These include the size and type of RF coil used for transmission, the distance of the coil from the patient, the field strength (B_0), and the number and type of RF pulses in the imaging sequence. For example, a 180° RF pulse requires four times the RF power of a 90° pulse, if the waveforms used are identical.

The rate at which energy (RF) is deposited into the body is defined as the specific absorption rate (SAR), measured in watts per kilogram body weight. The most recent Food and Drug Administration (FDA) guidelines (2003) limit RF power deposition to 4 W/kg averaged over 15 minutes for the whole body, 3 W/kg over 10 minutes for the head, 8 W/kg over 5 minutes per gram of tissue for the head or torso, and 12 W/kg over 5 minutes per gram of tissue for the extremities. Standards developed by the European Union (EU) differ, although with time the FDA and EU guidelines may be merged.

Metal, outside or inside the patient, may experience rapid and extreme heating due to applied RF, under certain circumstances. Reported incidents include first-, second-, and third-degree burns. Many of these incidents involved a part of the body being in direct contact with the RF coil used for transmission, or there were skin-to-skin contact points (a closed loop, with current flow possible within the body). Heating can occur due to current induction from the rapid switching of the gradients or from focused RF deposition. To prevent burns, there should be no unnecessary metal objects contacting the skin during the MR exam. Insulation (padding) should be used to prevent skin-to-skin contact points (closed loops). Insulating material (a minimum of 1 cm) should be placed between the patient's skin and the RF transmitter (often the body coil). Specific recommendations exist and should be followed for electrically conductive materials within the patient. For example, although MRI can be performed in a patient with a deep brain stimulator, this requires the utmost care. Failure to strictly follow safety recommendations can lead to serious permanent injury or even death. As such, it is important to monitor all patients during an MR exam— visually, verbally, and through the use of instruments such as a fiberoptic pulse oximeter.

$1 T = 42.6$ MHz

$1.5 T = 63$ MHz

5 Surface Coils

The closer the receiving antenna is to the source of the MR signal, the better the signal-to-noise ratio (SNR) will be. There are an impressive variety of coils available mainly to match the geometry and to allow optimal coverage of the different anatomic regions.

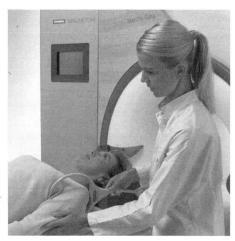

Figure 5–1

◆ Linearly Polarized (LP) Coils

A simple representation of a receiver antenna is a single conductive loop (Fig. **5–1**). The rotating magnetic moments cause a magnetic field fluctuation inside the loop area and, according to Maxwell's law, induce a voltage. The latter will be digitized and analyzed to provide the information necessary to create an image. To assign a rotating magnetic moment to the induced oscillating signal, the same signal is phase shifted by 90° and used as the "imaginary" part. That procedure is called "quadrature" detection.

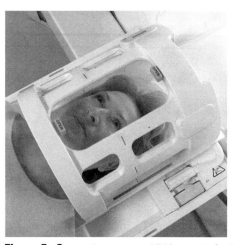

Figure 5–2

◆ Circularly Polarized (CP) Coils

Circularly polarized coils (Fig. **5–2**) are basically a combination of two linearly polarized coils that are arranged in such a way that they detect the rotation of the magnetic moments rather than just a linear field fluctuation. For example, the maximum signal detected by one coil is followed by a maximal signal detection in the adjacent coil arranged in the direction of the rotation of the magnetic moments. Because each coil is acquiring a new signal from the same source, the SNR improvement is about $\sqrt{2}$ as compared with an LP coil.

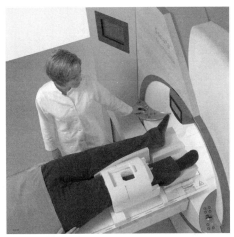

Figure 5–3

◆ Transmit/Receive and Receive Coils

Usually the body coil is the transmit coil creating an oscillating B_1 field of, for example, 2.3 μT for 2.5 ms to provide a 90° excitation pulse. For some applications, for example knee studies (Fig. **5–3**), it is beneficial to excite a smaller volume of interest. That requires less RF power as compared with a whole body excitation, and no signal will be generated from the adjacent anatomic structures, for example, the other knee, and no further actions will be necessary to avoid wraparound artifacts from those regions. Transmit coils are usually circularly polarized in design, because such coils require less power to provide a rotating B_1 field as compared with a linearly polarized coil.

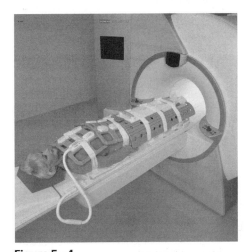

Figure 5–4

◆ CP Phased Array Coils

A small coil picks up less noise than a large coil, but may have only a limited coverage of the region of interest. The solution to this is simply to use more small coils. For multiple coils with multiple receiver channels and the utilization of circular polarization, the term *CP phased array* (Fig. **5–4**) has been established. Some vendors allow the combination of multiple CP phased array coils, for example, for the examination of different body parts that require different coverage in length as well as depth.

In addition to the larger coverage and the improved SNR due to sampling the same signal source independently with each coil, the geometrical arrangement of the coils contains some spatial information that can be used to reduce the number of encoding steps. Because the coils are acquiring the signal in parallel, those techniques are called "parallel acquisition" techniques.

6 Multichannel Coil Technology: Introduction

The increasing demand in MRI for large volumes of data with higher spatial resolution and a decrease in acquisition time requires the development and implementation of hardware that promotes the signal-to-noise ratio (SNR) and maximizes the efficiency of data handling. The SNR of an MR image is influenced by a variety of factors including the selected pulse sequence and magnet strength. However, the size of a signal receiving coil element, its proximity to the tissue being examined, and the number of RF receive channels also greatly affects the quality of an image and the time necessary to acquire it.

Early MR systems collected signal through linear polarized, single-element coils and transferred data to Fourier transform computers through one low bandwidth RF receive channel. Obtaining adequate SNR required that data be collected with lower imaging matrices and multiple signal averages leading to extended acquisition times. Additionally, because increasing the size of a single element has an inverse effect on the SNR, the volume of anatomic coverage was limited.

The introduction of circularly polarized (CP) coil structures led to a 40% increase in SNR through the use of two independent coil elements and allowed for greater anatomic coverage. However, with the demand for images with higher spatial resolution and the increased need for rapid data transfer in cases such as functional MR imaging, there remained room for improvement that called for greater efficiency in coil technology and RF channel hardware, leading to the development of multichannel technology. One application of current multichannel technology is illustrated in Fig. **6–1.** In this implementation, a coil containing eight elements is configured as a phased array with overlapping, circumferential coverage of the entire imaging volume, transferring signal through eight designated RF receive channels. Each of the individual coil elements acquires MR signals from the entire brain with the highest signal obtained from that portion of the tissue in closest proximity to the element. The small size of each element leads to a higher signal received from the adjacent tissue and a higher overall signal upon reconstruction. Fig. **6–2** illustrates the images acquired

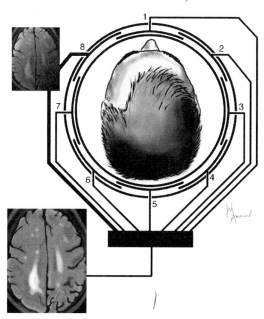

Figure 6–1

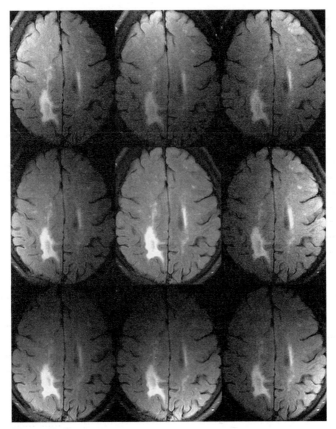

Figure 6–2

from each coil element, together with the final single combined image (in the middle) that is viewed by the radiologist. The scan illustrated is a fat-suppressed fluid-attenuated inversion recovery (FLAIR) from a patient with brain metastases, with the edema from a metastasis just superior and posterior to the lateral ventricles visualized.

Transferring the signal data through a reduced number of RF channels (as opposed to the full eight channels that compose this coil) would require that the information be combined through a method called multiplexing. However, this combining method causes an undesirable loss in signal and speed of transfer. For this reason, the signal from each element is transferred through a designated, high-bandwidth, RF channel allowing for faster transfer of large volumes of information, maintaining speed and signal. During reconstruction, the signal from each element is corrected to minimize element-to-element signal variations and then combined to form the final single image. Advanced reconstruction and storage hardware are also necessary to process the rapid inflow of information, reducing the limitations on data volume.

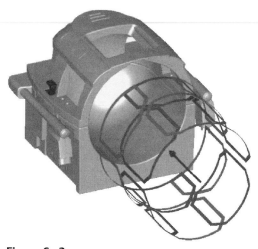

Figure 6–3

Fig. **6–3** demonstrates an example of a commercially available, 12-channel coil for brain imaging from Siemens Medical Solutions (Erlangen, Germany). Figs. **6–2** and **6–4** were acquired using an eight-channel coil from MRI Devices Corporation (Waukesha, WI).

MRI of the brain requires a good SNR and spatial resolution within an acceptable acquisition time. The higher SNR achieved with multichannel technology allows greater flexibility in sequence parameter selection including increased spatial resolution or reductions in acquisition time to minimize motion-induced artifacts.

The presented case demonstrates axial T1- and T2-weighted images of the brain at the level of the frontal horn of the right lateral ventricle and the sylvian fissure acquired with a standard circular polarized coil (Fig. **6–4A,C**) and an eight-element, phased array coil (Fig. **6–4B,D**). The MR system was equipped with eight high-bandwidth, RF receive channels to maximize the efficiency and speed of data transfer. Additionally, all pulse sequence parameters were held constant in the T1- as well as the T2-weighted examples to demonstrate the improvement in SNR. This demonstration shows clearly the benefit of multichannel technology in instances where reductions in scan time without a compromise in spatial resolution are necessary. The T1-weighted comparison demonstrates an appreciable increase in signal with corresponding reduction in noise from the eight-element coil, leading to an improved depiction of gray matter versus white matter in the cerebral cortex. An overall improvement in anatomic definition can be appreciated as well, illustrated by the improved visualization of cortical gyri and the sylvian fissure (Fig. **6–4B**). The SNR increase in the fast spin echo T2-weighted comparison is also reflected by the improved gray-white matter differentiation. There is improved definition of cortical gray matter, as well as improved visualization of the gray matter nuclei including the caudate head, globus pallidus, and putamen (Fig. **6–4D**).

Multichannel technology offers many additional benefits. Higher SNR provides the user with the ability to increase spatial resolution while maintaining acceptable levels of SNR, or combinations of increased spatial resolution and reduced scan time can be achieved. Additionally, applications collecting large amounts of information in a short time frame such as functional imaging benefit from higher SNR as well as faster data transfer and storage.

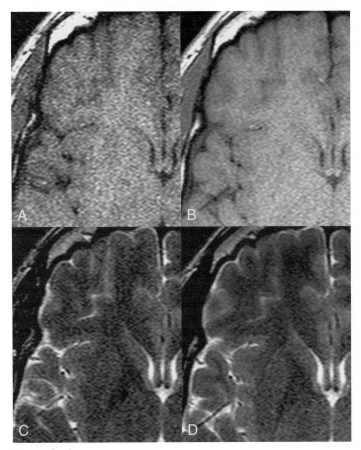

Figure 6 – 4

Advances in multielement/multichannel technology (to 32 elements and beyond) will continue to play a role in the development of imaging techniques with higher spatial resolution, faster scan times, and increased diagnostic quality of MR images.

7 Multichannel Coil Technology: Body Imaging

A major motivation for the introduction of surface coils (in the mid-1980s) was the reduction of background noise by limiting the sensitivity region of the coil to the volume of interest. A limited volume, unfortunately, also implied limited anatomic coverage. To compensate for this, combined surface coils or phased array coils were introduced. Further extension of this concept led to development of multichannel coil technology as we know it today. Illustrated in Fig. **7–1** is a 12-component coil, with six elements activated for acquisition of a single axial image. Each of the six numbered surface coils in the figure acquires signal from the anatomic region adjacent to the coil, with low sensitivity for noise outside the coil profile. The combined image takes advantage of the low sensitivity to noise and the high signal provided by each individual coil, the latter due to the close proximity to adjacent tissue. Thus, illustrated is parallel imaging using a multicoil multichannel system. The final composite image is color coded to show the dominant contribution in each sector from the nearest coil element.

Illustrated in Fig. **7–2,** arrayed around the periphery, are the individual images acquired by each of the six coil elements, with the final composite image in the center. The scan sequence employed was true fast imaging with steady-state precession (trueFISP), applied with spectral fat saturation, with two large liver hemangiomas well depicted. It should be noted that on current multichannel systems only the final

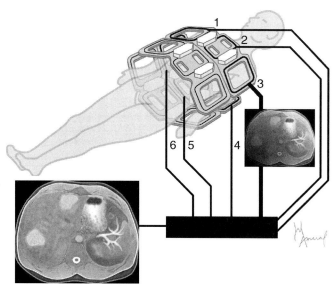

Figure 7–1   (see Color Plate 7–1, following page 130.)

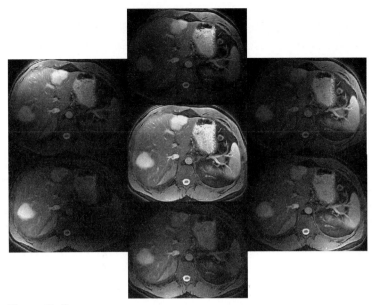

Figure 7 – 2

composite image is routinely provided for viewing, with the steps in between transparent to the user.

Apparent from Fig. **7 – 2,** and illustrated in Fig. **7 – 3,** is the spatial information that is contained in the coil sensitivity profile. The coarse structure of an object, which is commonly acquired with a low phase-encoding step, can be derived from the coil sensitivity profile. The only prerequisite is that the sensitivity profiles of multiple coils have to extend in the direction of phase encoding. Fig. **7 – 3** illustrates the replacement of spatial information, acquired with a phase encoding step in conventional imaging, with spatial information provided by the coil sensitivity profile.

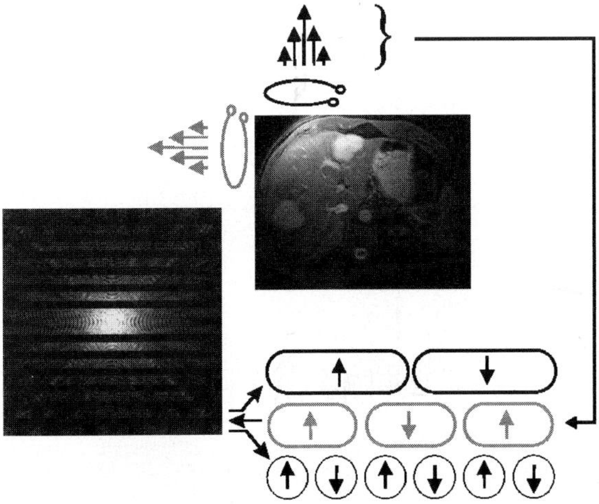

Dynamic imaging of the heart is commonly performed with a balanced gradient echo technique, acquiring multiple Fourier lines per heart phase per cardiac cycle, to allow data sampling in a breath hold period.

The utilization of a parallel acquisition technique using multiple coils will allow a reduction in the number of Fourier lines to be measured, while still maintaining the matrix size and therefore the spatial resolution.

Figure 7 – 3

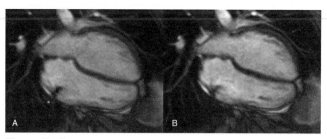

Figure 7 – 4

Fig. **7 – 4** shows a single four-chamber view of a bright blood dynamic acquisition. Fig. **7 – 4A** was acquired with a measurement protocol lasting seven heartbeats. Fig. **7 – 4B** is based on the same protocol but with the use of a parallel acquisition factor of 2, leading to a reduction in measurement time to four heartbeats.

It has to be kept in mind that each measured Fourier line is considered an additional acquisition, because each Fourier line contains information from the whole object. Omitting the measurement of Fourier lines will not only lead to artifacts, but will also reduce the overall signal-to-noise ratio (SNR) of the measurement. The artifacts will be taken care of using the spatial information contained in the sensitivity profiles of the surface coils. The drop in SNR is something that is typical for parallel acquisition techniques. Use of parallel imaging, specifically for replacement of Fourier lines, is only feasible in applications that provide sufficient SNR. Fig. **7 – 5** presents images from a bright blood dynamic imaging acquisition using a balanced gradient echo imaging technique, providing a short axis view of the right and left ventricular chambers. Fig. **7 – 5A** was acquired during four heart beats, whereas Fig. **7 – 5B** represents a breath hold acquisition requiring only three heart beats.

Morphologic images of the heart are mostly acquired with a fast spin echo acquisition scheme with a preceding preparation leading to a hypointense appearance of blood. Keeping the echo train length constant but reducing the number of Fourier lines that need to be acquired by utilizing parallel acquisition techniques with a multiple coil arrangement will lead to a reduction in measurement time. Fig. **7 – 6** presents four chamber (Fig. **7 – 6A, B**) and short axis views (Fig. **7 – 6C, D**) acquired with a "dark blood" fast spin echo acquisition for a measurement acquisition lasting

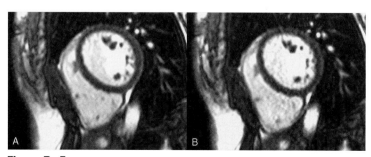

Figure 7 – 5

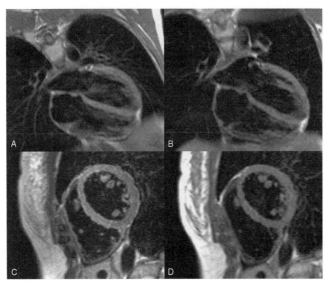

Figure 7 – 6

14 heart beats (no parallel acquisition technique) (Fig. **7 – 6A, C**) versus images acquired in a breath hold period of eight heart beats utilizing a parallel acquisition factor of two (Fig. **7 – 6B, D**).

Axial images through the liver and gallbladder, acquired with fast spin echo technique and spectral fat saturation, are illustrated in Fig. **7 – 7**. With the introduction of fast spin echo imaging, breath-hold T2-weighted abdominal scans became feasible. Parallel imaging can be used to further reduce scan time, a common current application. Alternatively, with fast spin echo technique, parallel imaging can be used to reduce the echo train length while keeping scan time the same. One advantage of using a shorter echo train is that more slices can be acquired within the same scan time. Fig. **7 – 7A** is an example of a 17-second T2-weighted breath hold acquisition. Whereas 29 echoes were used to acquire the data for Fig. **7 – 7A**, only 19 echoes were used to acquire the data for Fig. **7 – 7B**. Fig. **7 – 7B** represents an identical acquisition with the same measurement duration but reduced echo train length. The missing Fourier lines for Fig. **7 – 7B** were reconstructed using parallel imaging.

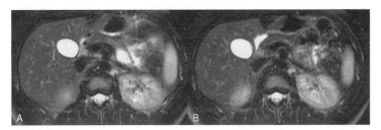

Figure 7 – 7

8 Triggering and Gating: Functional Imaging

Although there are several imaging protocols available to collect an image in a time shorter than a heart beat, a longer imaging protocol may be required to achieve sufficient spatial resolution or adequate signal-to-noise ratio (SNR). For the beating heart or organs within the abdomen that change location during respiration, it may be necessary to trigger or gate the image acquisition using some type of physiologic monitoring. Monitoring of the heartbeat can be done using either the ECG signal or a pulse sensor (attached to a finger).

◆ Prospective Triggering (ECG)

In prospective ECG triggering, image acquisition starts with the detection of the QRS complex. As an example, for a short TR gradient echo sequence, multiple images of the same slice can be generated by acquiring data during small time windows within the cardiac cycle. The common approach is to measure multiple Fourier lines per heart beat as illustrated in Fig. **8–1.** The number of heart beats necessary to acquire the image data are equal to the number of required phase-encoding steps divided by the number of Fourier-lines measured per heart beat. The acquisition of more than one Fourier line per heart beat for the same image (of the point in time within the cardiac cycle) is sometimes referred to as "segmented" scanning. The temporal resolution is given by the time it takes to acquire the number of Fourier lines per heart beat (a "segment"). Temporal resolution can be improved by measuring the center of k space more often, using the high spatial frequency information from adjacent measurement windows to get another full k-space matrix for the calculation of an additional image. This method is called echo sharing or view sharing.

The images of the "four chamber view" of the heart in Fig. **8–1** were acquired using a gradient echo (GRE) fast low-angle shot (FLASH) sequence, where the contrast between blood and myocardium relies on the inflow of unsaturated blood. Matrix size and segmentation has been adjusted to achieve a measurement time of 15 heartbeats, short enough to allow a breath-hold acquisition. Fig. **8–1A** shows the four-chamber view in end diastole. At this point in time there is a high contrast between blood and myocardial wall due to the inflow effect of unsaturated blood. Fig. **8–1B** shows the same view at end systole. The mitral valve is still closed and the blood in the left ventricle is saturated, whereas the left atrium has already received unsaturated blood. The image shown in Fig. **8–1C** was acquired at the beginning of diastole, where the mitral valve is open and the unsaturated blood is flowing from the left atrium into the left ventricle.

Some prospective triggered studies continue to apply RF pulses during the remaining part of end diastole without the collection of any data, just to keep the

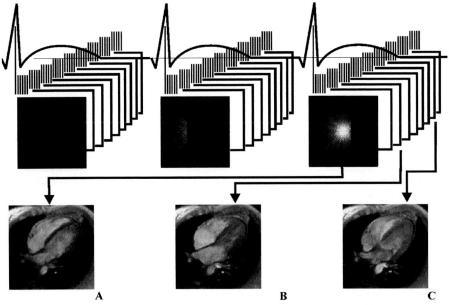

Figure 8–1

signal response at the same level to achieve an identical image appearance for all phases of the cardiac cycle. If the RF excitation is applied only during imaging, the longitudinal magnetization will have more time to recover between the last image acquired in end diastole and the first image acquired at the beginning of systole, leading to a different contrast for the first image as compared with all other images of the cardiac cycle. Prospectively triggered acquisitions also have the disadvantage that they do not cover the complete cardiac cycle. There is always a part of end diastole, just before the next detected QRS complex, that is going to be missed.

Prospective triggering is also used to acquire T1- or T2-weighted images using a fast spin echo scheme. A common approach is to perform a "dark blood" preparation at the time the QRS complex is detected and to acquire the Fourier lines during end diastole, where the motion of the heart is reduced.

◆ Prospective Triggering (Pulse Sensor)

The signal from a pulse monitor can be used as an alternative to trigger events that are correlated with arterial pulsation (Fig. **8–2**). It has to be noted, however, that the associated cardiac event is already history. Due to slight variations in heart rate, recorded cardiac events using a pulse trigger will result in slightly blurred images of the heart.

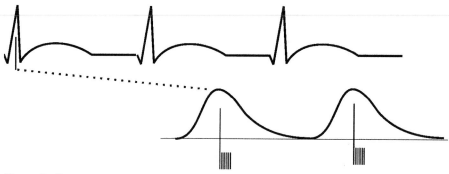

Figure 8 – 2

◆ Retrospective Cardiac Gating

With retrospective cardiac gating (Fig. **8 – 3**), identical Fourier lines are acquired for a user-defined duration, or, if several adjacent Fourier lines are measured, a specific portion of the k space is measured in that time. Each Fourier line or k-space segment is given a time stamp relative to the most recently detected QRS complex. Once all k-space segments have been acquired, the Fourier lines are sorted into as many k-space matrices (images) per cardiac cycle, as the user defined.

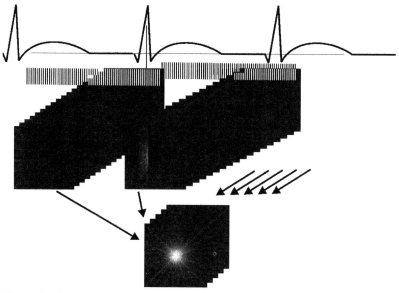

Figure 8 – 3

Uma Vakcti, MD

◆ Arrhythmia Rejection

Some imaging protocols allow the option of arrhythmia rejection, in which case the system will monitor the average duration of the cardiac cycle and will retrospectively reject the data acquired during an abnormally short or long cardiac cycle (Fig. **8–4**). The system will also take note that the rejected data still have to be acquired.

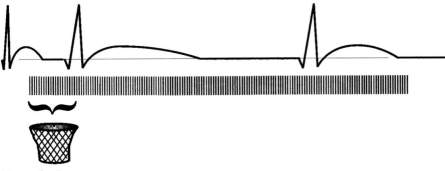

Figure 8–4

◆ External Trigger

Similar to the ECG trigger, most systems allow connection to an external trigger device for initiation of the imaging sequence (Fig. **8–5**). In the future it may no longer be necessary to use trigger devices, because the MR signal itself contains information about motion ("self-gating").

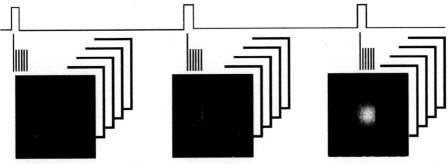

Figure 8–5

9 Triggering: Morphologic Imaging

◆ Morphologic Imaging (Dark Blood)

For the assessment of cardiac morphology, "dark blood" pulse sequences were developed and are in widespread use. Following the detection of a QRS complex, a nonselective inversion pulse is applied, immediately followed by a selective "reinversion" pulse for the slice to be imaged (Fig. **9–1**). During a waiting period, the reinverted blood is washed out of the imaging slice and is replaced by inverted blood. Image

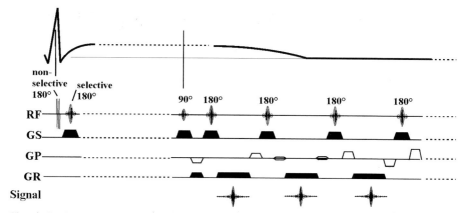

Figure 9–1

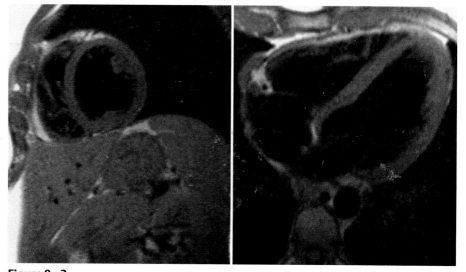

Figure 9–2

acquisition follows, using either a fast spin echo or segmented gradient echo sequence, resulting in a "dark blood" image. Data acquisition for morphologic imaging is performed preferably in diastole, to avoid the rapid movements of the contracting heart in systole. Fig. **9-2** shows short and long axis images of the heart acquired using a "dark blood" fast spin echo sequence. This approach, applied with high resolution and fat saturation, is used as an adjunct in protocols screening for dysrhythmogenic right ventricular dysplasia (in which there is thinning and replacement of muscle by fatty or fibrous tissue, with enlargement of the ventricle at end diastole).

◆ Respiratory Triggering

The signal from a respiratory belt (Fig. **9-3**) can be used to initiate an imaging sequence at a specified time within the respiratory cycle. Triggering is user-defined based on a threshold, while monitoring the signal pattern coming from the respiratory belt (Fig. **9-4**). The trigger point is set to be close to either end-inspiration or end-expiration. Sequences that rely on a steady-state signal are usually continuously applied without collecting the signal data. In this case, data acquisition is initiated after the "trigger" point has been passed. Fig. **9-5A** is an example of a gradient echo image acquisition during free breathing. Fig. **9-5B** shows the same slice acquired using free breathing, but with data acquisition triggered by the signal from the respiratory belt (20% threshold prior to reaching end-expiration). Note the marked reduction in blurring.

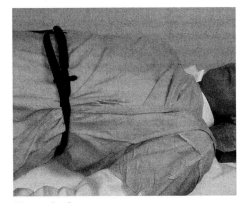

Figure 9-3

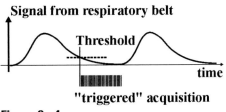

Figure 9-4

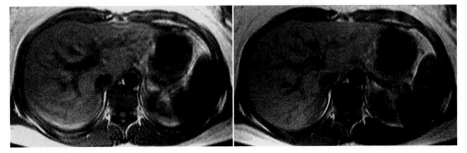

Figure 9-5

10 Imaging Basics: k Space, Raw Data, Image Data

The signal for MRI comes from the nuclei of hydrogen. Because the hydrogen nucleus consists of a single proton, it is common practice to refer to the signal as coming from protons. On exposing the patient to a magnetic field, more nuclear magnetic moments (of protons) will be aligned with (parallel to) the main magnetic field rather than against it. This results in a net longitudinal magnetization. Tilting of that magnetization can be done with an RF pulse. Once the magnetization is tilted away from the parallel alignment, it will start to precess around the direction of the main magnetic field with the Larmor frequency. That frequency is a function of the local magnetic field strength. To tilt the magnetization, the frequency of the RF pulse must match the rotational frequency of that magnetization. Establishing a magnetic field gradient along the direction of slice selection (e.g., z) and using an RF pulse with a limited frequency range will result in a slice-selective excitation (Fig. **10–1**). Magnetizations of different resonance frequencies remain untouched. Following a 90° RF pulse, the longitudinal magnetization is converted into transverse magnetization. The latter is responsible for the observed MR signal and will be encoded with spatial information.

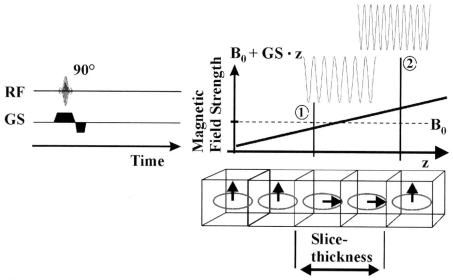

Figure 10–1

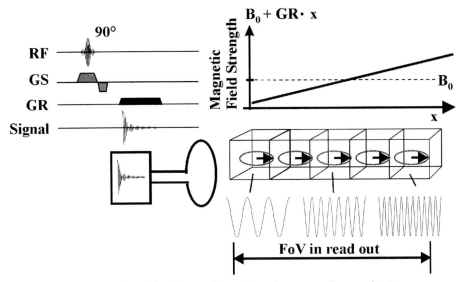

Figure 10–2 GS = slice-selective gradient; GP = phase encoding gradient; GR = readout gradient.

Fig. **10–1** is an illustration of a slice-selective excitation utilizing the dependency of resonance frequencies on local magnetic field strength; (1) and (2) mark the lower and upper frequency range covered with the slice-selective RF pulse. Essential to spatial encoding in MRI is the fact that the resonance frequency of the magnetization is a function of the local magnetic field strength. Establishing a magnetic field gradient across an object (e.g., B_0 + GR * x) will result in different frequencies along that direction (e.g., x) (Fig. **10–2**).

Fig. **10–2** is an illustration of frequency encoding by means of a magnetic field gradient. The rotating transverse magnetizations induce a MR signal in an adjacent coil. The signal decays rapidly due to fast dephasing based on the different frequencies. The magnetic field gradient is encoding via frequencies and is called the frequency-encoding gradient. An alternative term is the readout gradient (GR), because the gradient is on during readout of the data. The frequency-encoding gradient spreads the Larmor frequency over a sufficiently wide range to distinguish the individual voxels specified in that direction. An adjacent RF receiver coil will see one transverse magnetization being the sum of all transverse magnetizations of each individual voxel. The range of different frequencies causes a rapid dephasing of the transverse magnetization, resulting in the induced signal rapidly decaying. The algorithm used to analyze the frequency contributions (Fourier transformation) differentiates the contribution of adjacent voxels if the transverse magnetization of those adjacent voxels is of opposite sign at the beginning and at the end of the data chain. This can be achieved by switching on a negative GR of half the duration of the data acquisition window prior to data acquisition (Fig. **10–3**).

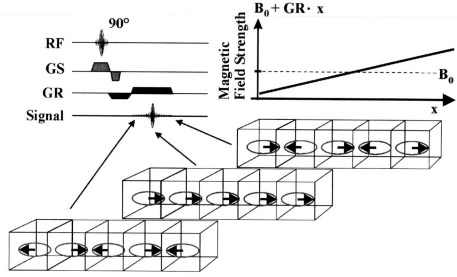

Figure 10 – 3

Analyzing the received signal for frequency contributions is called a Fourier transformation. The amplitude of the contribution is assigned to a pixel intensity at the location of the measured frequency (Fig. **10 – 4**).

The signal course is called an echo, and because gradient switching has been used it is called a gradient echo (GRE). The algorithm (fast Fourier transformation, FFT) analyzes the collected data for frequency contributions. Because the spatial

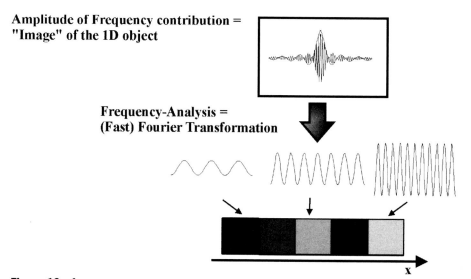

Figure 10 – 4

distribution of frequencies is known (dictated by the magnetic field gradient applied), the FFT can assign the amplitude of the different frequency contributions to specific locations, in this example the location of a one-dimensional (1D) object (Fig. **10–4**).

The data acquired during one readout period is called a Fourier line. Because each data point along the line has an index referred to as a "k" value in mathematics, the line is also called a k-space line. For 2D-encoding the single Fourier line is expanded to a Fourier space or k space. The data structure in the second dimension is similar to the data structure along a Fourier line. The high spatial frequencies are contained at the beginning and at the end of a Fourier line, where the magnetizations of adjacent voxels will have opposite signs. Similar phase positions are encoded in the phase-encoding direction. The first Fourier and the last Fourier k-space lines correspond to the situation in which adjacent voxels in the phase-encoding direction have opposite signs. For an unambiguous assignment of locations, the measurement has to be repeated with lower phase encoding amplitudes to sample the coarse structure of the object. All magnetizations point in one direction at the center of k space.

The number of data points taken in either direction (GR and GP) has to be equal to or larger than the matrix resolution of the image to unambiguously assign the signal to a location. For example, a 256 by 512 image resolution requires that at least 256 phase-encoding steps are acquired and 512 data points are sampled during the readout period. If fewer Fourier lines are measured, as in half Fourier or parallel imaging techniques, additional algorithms have to supplement the missing information. The important message is that the center of k space contains nothing other than the information of how much signal the whole excited slice is sending (Fig. **10–5**). Adjacent to the center of k space in either direction is the information about the coarse structures of the objects within the slice. The information about the requested highest resolution is found in the outer borders of k space. The spatial resolution is given by the selected field of view (FOV) divided by the matrix size in either direction. The first and last Fourier lines within the k space for each slice excited corresponds to a situation where all magnetic moments in the adjacent voxel within one slice in the direction of GP point in opposite directions [(iii) and (iv)].

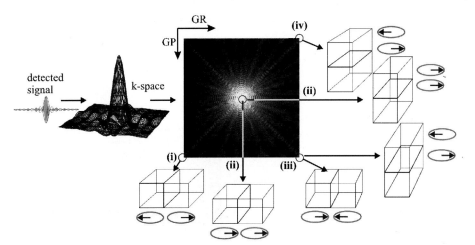

Figure 10–5

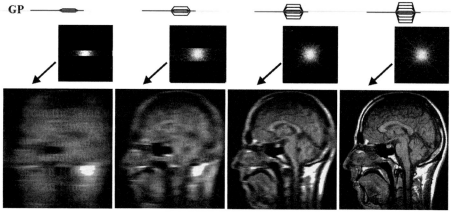

Figure 10 – 6

In addition, the first and last data points of each Fourier line represent the situation also that adjacent voxels in the direction of GR have opposite directions for the transverse magnetization [(i) and (iii)]. The center of k space contains the maximum signal with all transverse magnetizations of the excited slice pointing in the same direction (ii).

Fig. **10 – 6** illustrates how the spatial resolution gradually improves with increasing numbers of Fourier lines around the center of k space.

For all imaging sequences, the data structure is identical for the frequency encoding and the phase encoding directions. The change in phase position during data sampling in the presence of a frequency encoding gradient will later allow the identification of the frequency contribution. The same change in phase position in the direction of the phase encoding gradient is later analyzed to identify the origin of the signal.

To summarize a measurement (Fig. **10 – 7**):

1. A slice-selective gradient is established in the direction of slice selection (GS, e.g., z).

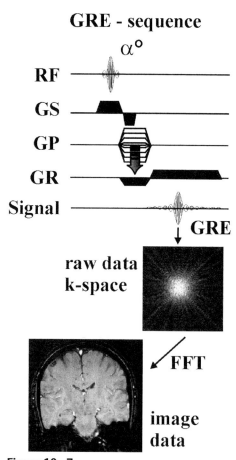

Figure 10 – 7

2. Once that gradient is established an RF excitation pulse will excite the slice, i.e., it will tilt the longitudinal magnetization to become transverse magnetization.

3. A phase encoding gradient, GP, will establish partial spatial information in the direction of the gradient.

4. A readout gradient, GR, will be activated to prepare the starting point for the first data point (transverse magnetization of adjacent voxels to point in opposite directions). During data acquisition, GR is switched on, creating a gradient echo (GRE) with a signal maximum close to the center of k space. A 2D Fourier transformation (2D FFT) will assign pixel intensities within the image based on a 2D frequency analysis. For the advanced reader, some of the stated prerequisites are not mandatory. For example, it is common in GRE techniques to shift the echo center to the earlier time in k space. The signal will be stronger due to the shorter TE, with the artifacts caused by the k-space asymmetry outweighed by that benefit.

11 Image Resolution: Pixel and Voxel Size

MRI spatial resolution, the ability to distinguish structures as separate and distinct from each other, is inherently related to the acquired voxel volume. The field of view (FOV), acquisition matrix, and the slice thickness determine voxel volume. The pixel size (FOV/matrix) determines the in-plane resolution. Reducing the FOV, increasing the matrix number, or reducing the slice thickness results in an image with reduced voxel volume. Small voxels produce MR images with high spatial resolution but lower signal-to-noise ratio (SNR), and thus may appear somewhat "grainy" compared with images acquired with a larger voxel volume.

The images shown in Fig. **11–1** demonstrate the effect of altering the pixel and/or voxel size. All are T1-weighted images. Fig. **11–1A** and **11–1C** were acquired using a matrix of 128 × 128, and Fig. **11–1B** and **11–1D** with a matrix of 256 × 256. The 256 × 256 images have higher spatial resolution but lower SNR. In addition, a truncation artifact is visible in Fig. **11–1C** (arrow) due to the reduced matrix in the phase encoding direction (right to left). To summarize, reducing the pixel size increases spatial resolution but reduces SNR (assuming all other factors are held constant).

The images in Fig. **11–1E** and **11–1F** were acquired using a three-dimensional (3D) scan technique with heavy T1-weighting. A 3D acquisition excites an entire slab or volume of tissue rather than a slice. The slices are produced by the application of an additional phase encoding gradient in the slice (z) direction. In a conventional steady-state 3D sequence, the number of slices (sometimes referred to as "partitions") desired determines the number of phase encoding steps to be applied in the slice direction and thus directly affects scan time. Fig. **11–1E** is one slice from a 3D data set acquired with a slice thickness of 2 mm, whereas Fig. **11–1F** was acquired with a thickness of 1 mm. The 1-mm partition demonstrates higher spatial resolution but lower SNR than the 2-mm partition. 3D acquisitions are useful for acquiring thin contiguous slices with high SNR. In addition, reformatted images from a 3D data set (for example in the sagittal and coronal planes) will be of high quality if the voxel dimensions are near isotropic (equal in all three dimensions).

SNR in MR can be a very complicated subject. But it is simply the signal divided by the noise in an image. Looking only at image resolution and matrix size, the signal is directly proportional to the acquisition voxel volume. The noise is proportional to the inverse of the square root of the number of 2D phase encoding steps times the number of 3D phase encoding steps.

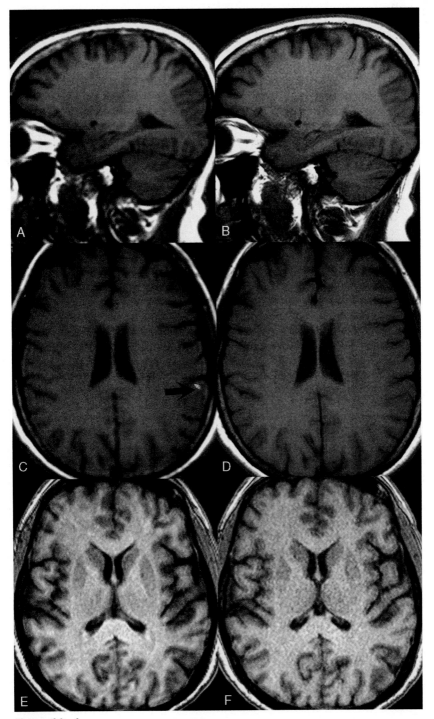

Figure 11 – 1

12 Imaging Basics: Signal-to-Noise Ratio (SNR)

The images in this case illustrate the critical concept of signal-to-noise ratio (SNR) in MR. SNR, as the term implies, is the ratio of MR signal to noise, specifically for the spatially encoded voxel. MR images acquired with a low SNR appear somewhat "grainy" to the eye (Fig. **12–1A,C**) especially when compared with images acquired with higher SNR (Fig. **12–1B,D**). It is important to note that the human eye does not perceive SNR per se but rather the contrast-to-noise ratio (CNR). The higher the contrast between two structures, the less SNR required to visualize the difference between the two structures. For example, the difference between gray and white matter is much easier to see in Fig. **12–1B** (with higher SNR) than in Fig. **12–1A**.

Let us first consider what determines the signal in a spatially encoded voxel. MR signal is directly proportional to the size of the voxel. The larger the voxel, the greater the number of hydrogen protons and thus the greater the MR signal. Larger voxels, however, result in reduced spatial resolution (see case 11). The parameters that affect the size of the voxel in a 2D acquisition are field of view (FOV), the number of phase encoding steps (acquired phase encoding matrix), the number of frequency encoding steps (acquired frequency or read matrix), and the slice thickness. As stated, SNR is directly proportional to the size of the voxel. So, for example, doubling the slice thickness will double the voxel volume and double SNR. However, the FOV affects the voxel volume in two dimensions. As such, reducing the FOV by a factor of 2 would reduce the voxel volume and SNR by a factor of 4.

Turning to a consideration of noise, the noise in a voxel is equal to the square root of the sampling bandwidth (an operator-defined variable) for the voxel divided by the square root of the total number of times the voxel is sampled. The parameters that affect the number of times the voxel is sampled, and thus the noise in the voxel, are the number of phase encoding steps, the number of slices encoded (for a 3D acquisition only), and the number of signals averaged (NSA). NSA is the number of times each line of k space is sampled and is also known as the number of excitations (NEX) or acquisitions, depending on vendor. NSA is the parameter most often increased in the clinical setting to increase SNR. The problem with increasing NSA to increase SNR (in this case by reducing the noise) is that that the total scan time is directly related to the NSA while the SNR is related to the square root of the change in NSA. For example, if NSA (and thus scan time) is increased by a factor of 4 (the difference in Fig. **12–1** between **A** and **B,** and likewise between **C** and **D**), SNR will only increase by a factor of the square root of 4 (and thus 2).

As noted, SNR is also inversely proportional to the square root of the sampling (receiver) bandwidth of the encoded voxel. For example, if one were to reduce the receiver bandwidth by a factor of 2, SNR would increase by a factor of the square root of 2. While receiver bandwidth does not affect scan time, reducing the receiver bandwidth does increase chemical shift artifact (see case 96), which can be more problematic at higher field strengths.

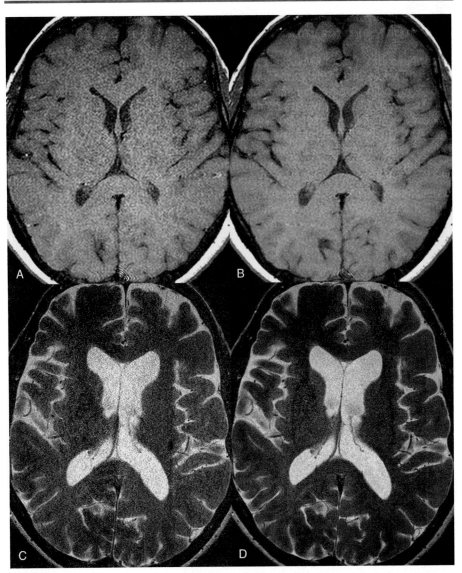

Figure 12–1

13 Imaging Basics: Contrast-to-Noise Ratio (CNR)

The contrast-to-noise ratio (CNR) is defined as the difference in signal contribution (signal intensity, SI) between different tissues, divided by the background noise (N).

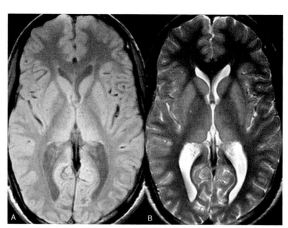

Figure 13–1

For example, the contrast between cerebrospinal fluid (CSF) and white matter (WM) is given by $(SI_{CSF} - SI_{WM})/N$. Fig. **13–1** demonstrates the improved CNR achieved for proton density (PD) weighted scans with (**B**) fast spin echo (FSE) as opposed to (**A**) spin echo (SE) technique (**A** and **B** are from a normal volunteer). The TR of 2.8 seconds used with the SE sequence is too short for true proton density weighting, providing hypointense CSF due to the fact that the longitudinal magnetization of CSF is still not fully recovered. With FSE, scan times can be significantly shorter despite the use of a longer TR (5.6 seconds in this instance), leading to hyperintense signal from CSF, as one would expect due to the higher proton density within CSF as compared with gray and white matter. Scan time for the SE images was 11.6 minutes, as opposed to 2.1 minutes for the FSE images. The contrast-to-noise ratio between gray and white matter is also improved with FSE imaging, due not to the choice of TR and TE but to magnetization transfer effects from the multiple 180° RF pulses. Fig. **13–2A,B** presents a similar comparison, (**A**) SE vs. (**B**) FSE, in a patient with multiple sclerosis (MS). Although CSF is higher signal intensity on the FSE image, the CNR between the MS plaque (arrow) along the right lateral ventricle and adjacent CSF is actually lower.

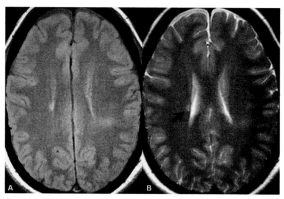

Figure 13–2

14 SNR Versus CNR

Fig. **14–1A,C** depicts the signal-to-noise ratio (SNR) for white (WM) and gray matter (GM), and their contrast-to-noise ratio (CNR) for identical measurement times but different TR values. Scan time was held constant, despite TR being twice as long, by using two acquisitions (averages) for the first scan. Increasing the TR from 430 ms (Fig. **14–1B**) to 860 ms (Fig. **14–1D**) on a 1.5 T system will lead to a ~7% increase in SNR for WM, but a ~30% drop in CNR (WM/GM)! Selecting a TR of 860 ms will increase the overall signal from both GM and WM, but the CNR will be significantly lower. Visualization of both the edema and normal gray-white matter differentiation (arrows) in this example is improved with the shorter TR (higher CNR).

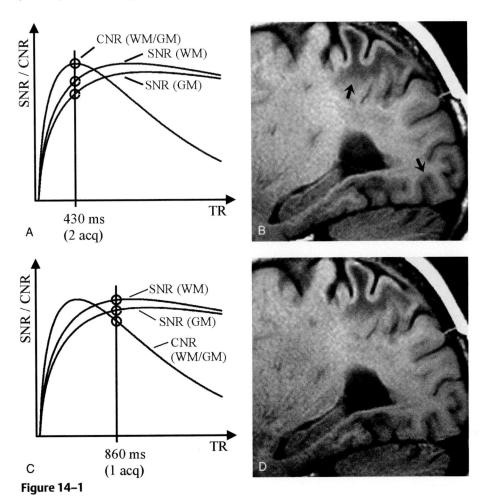

Figure 14–1

15 T1, T2, and Proton Density

When imaging with computed tomography (CT), there is only one intrinsic contrast mechanism, and that is the electron density of the tissues being examined. Also, with CT, one does not adjust any extrinsic contrast parameters in that the kilovolts (kV) used remains high. This is not the case, however, with MRI.

There are many intrinsic contrast mechanisms that one can utilize in MRI. The ones discussed in this chapter include proton (spin) density (PD), T1 relaxation time, and T2 relaxation time. Images are usually acquired for which the contrast is weighted more toward one of these parameters. The key word here is "weighted." Tissue contrast in the image has contributions from each of the various intrinsic contrast mechanisms, but is "weighted" more toward one than the others. In this context, weighting simply means the amount of contribution made to the image contrast associated with the difference between tissues on the basis of the parameter of interest (PD, T1, or T2). This weighting is accomplished by the selection of the timing parameters of the pulse sequence (set prior to scan acquisition). For spin echo sequences, these are the TR (repetition time) and the TE (echo time).

TR primarily controls the amount of T1-weighting, whereas TE primarily controls the amount of T2-weighting. If one wishes to obtain images in which the contrast is weighted more toward T1, then a relatively short TR is selected. There is no exact "best" TR, but rather a range to produce T1-weighted images. The range depends on the tissues being imaged as well as the field strength of the MR system. T1 relaxation times decrease as field strength is reduced and increase (lengthen) as field strength increases. At 1.5 T, when acquiring T1-weighted images of the brain (Fig. **15–1A**), the TR is usually between 400 and 550 ms. Raising the TR will not make the image more T2-weighted, but rather simply reduce the T1-weighting.

As previously mentioned, TE primarily controls the amount of T2-weighting in an MR image. If one desires a T1-weighted image, a relatively short TE is selected. Often, one selects the shortest TE possible. For spin echo images, short is 25 ms or less. If one desires a T2-weighted image, then the TR is increased to reduce the amount of T1-weighting (usually 2500 ms or higher), and a long TE is selected. For spin echo, this is usually 80 to 120 ms. Fig. **15–1B** is an example of a T2-weighted spin echo image (long TR/long TE).

To obtain proton density weighted images (Fig. **15–1C**), one increases the TR to reduce the T1-weighting (again to $\geq$ 2500 ms) and reduces the TE (to 25 ms or less) to reduce the T2-weighting. Although one may choose to acquire PD-weighted images, in clinical practice however, T2-weighted fluid-attenuated inversion recovery (FLAIR) sequences (Fig. **15–1D**) have supplanted proton density weighted scans for imaging of the brain.

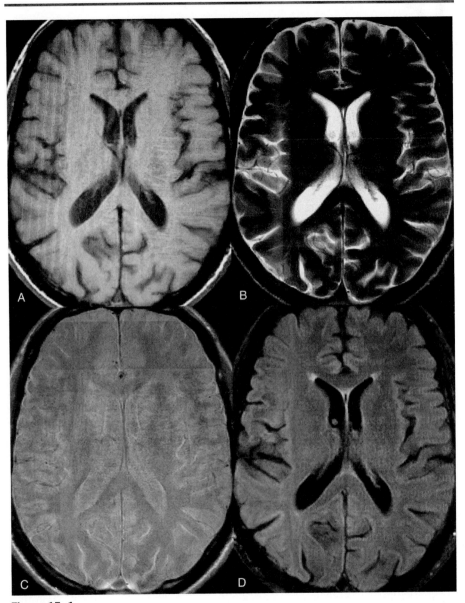

Figure 15–1

16 Spin Echo Imaging

Sagittal and axial T1-weighted spin echo images are shown prior to (Fig. **16–1A,C**) and coronal and axial images following (Fig. **16–1B,D**) intravenous gadolinium chelate administration. The scans demonstrate a heterogeneously enhancing mass in the left parietooccipital region, which at surgery was documented to be a glioblastoma multiforme.

In an MR pulse sequence, an echo (which constitutes the observed signal) is formed by either a refocusing gradient magnetic field alone or with an RF pulse prior to the echo. A sequence that uses a gradient only to refocus the echo is referred to as a "gradient echo" pulse sequence. If there is an RF pulse prior to the echo (generally a 180° pulse), then the pulse sequence is referred to as a "spin echo" sequence. Spin echo (SE) imaging has historically been the "workhorse" pulse sequence of clinical MRI.

In a spin echo pulse sequence, the 90° RF pulse (the first pulse applied) produces transverse magnetization (tipping the net vector from parallel to the field into the transverse plane). This induces a signal in the receiver coil known as the free induction decay (FID). A 180° RF pulse is then applied and the echo formed at the time TE (the time between the initial 90° pulse and the echo). The time between the 90° and 180° pulse is often referred to as tau and is equal to TE/2. The 180° RF pulse also corrects for dephasing effects from field and local inhomogeneities as well as chemical shift effects one sees when fat and water are located within a single voxel. Therefore, using a spin echo pulse sequence, the image contrast, based on the TE selected, is dependent on T2 (the spin-spin or transverse relaxation time) rather than T2* (the effective spin-spin relaxation time, which is faster than T2 because it includes the effects of static field inhomogeneities).

There are two operator-selectable timing parameters, which can be varied to control the contrast of the image when using SE sequences. These parameters are TR (repetition time) and TE (echo time). The TR determines the T1-weighting and the TE determines the T2-weighting. As discussed in case 15, the use of a relatively short TR (i.e., 500 ms or less) and a short TE (i.e., 25 ms or less) produces images in which the tissue contrast is primarily related to differences in T1-relaxation times. Tissues with short T1 relaxation times appear bright on T1-weighted images. Gadolinium is a paramagnetic metal and, when in close proximity to a water molecule, the paramagnetic effect shortens the T1 of the water protons resulting in high signal intensity on T1-weighted images (Fig. **16–1B,D**).

Increasing the TR while maintaining a short TE produces images that are primarily proton density weighted. Using a long TR (>2000 ms) and a long TE (>80 ms) produces images that are T2-weighted. Because increasing TR also increases scan time, proton density and T2-weighted scans are now acquired using fast spin echo technique, as opposed to traditional spin echo technique (see case 17).

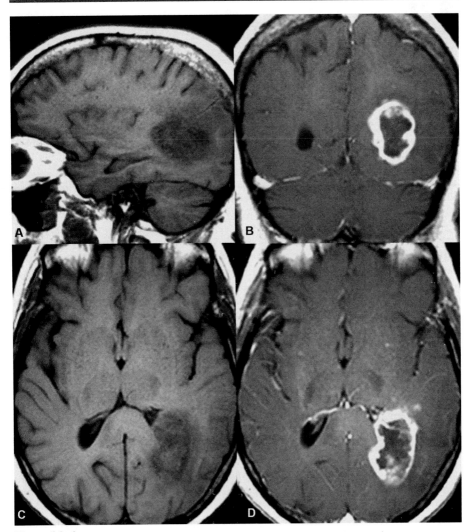

Figure 16–1

Given that TR in a SE sequence is much longer than TE, SE scans are performed in a multislice fashion. During the time following the echo, other slices are excited. The maximum number of slices one can acquire during a given pulse sequence is dependent primarily on TR/TE. Reducing the TR or increasing the TE reduces the number of slices one can acquire for a given SE pulse sequence.

17 Fast Spin Echo Imaging

The images illustrated were acquired using conventional spin echo (Fig. **17–1A,B**) and fast spin echo (Fig. **17–1C,D**) techniques. The use of fast spin echo (FSE) imaging has become routine in MRI today. A spin echo sequence employs a 180° RF pulse to create the echo, which also corrects for dephasing effects from slight field inhomogeneities and chemical shift. In a conventional spin echo sequence, a phase encoding gradient of defined amplitude is applied prior to the collection of the echo during readout. The amplitude of the phase encoding gradient determines the line in k space that will be filled as the echo is sampled. In a conventional spin echo sequence, one line of k space is filled during each repetition (TR period) of the pulse sequence. In an FSE sequence, a series of 180° pulses produces a train of echoes during a single TR period. The number of echoes produced in a single TR period is known as the echo train length (ETL). The phase encoding gradient amplitude will vary prior to each echo in the train so that each echo will fill a different line of k space. In this way, multiple lines of k space are filled during a single TR period. The number of lines filled in a single TR thus also corresponds to the ETL. As an example, using an ETL of 16, 16 lines of k space will be filled during a single TR period. If a phase encoding matrix of 256 is selected, rather than requiring 256 repetitions of the pulse sequence to fill all the lines of k space [assuming 1 for the number of signals averaged (NSA)], only 16 repetitions would be required (256/16 = 16). Increasing the ETL to 32 would require only eight repetitions to fill all 256 lines of k space. The use of FSE sequences has not only greatly reduced the time required to obtain MR images with a long TR, but allows the use of high TR times for improved tissue contrast.

To demonstrate the power of FSE, consider the images in Fig. **17–1A,B**. They were acquired using conventional spin echo technique with a TR of 3500 ms and a TE of 85 ms. The total scan time was 10 minutes, 51 seconds. The FSE sequence (Fig. **17–1C,D**) was acquired using the same TR and TE but it had an ETL of 19. By filling 19 lines of k space in each TR period, the scan time for the FSE images was only 35 seconds (10:51 divided by 19). The multiple 180° pulses also help reduce pulsation and flow artifacts. Note the higher cerebrospinal fluid (CSF) signal intensity around the pons and improved depiction of flow voids in the basilar and internal carotid arteries in the FSE images, together with reduced ghosting from CSF, vessels, and the globes.

As previously mentioned, increasing the ETL reduces scan time; however, this is not without penalty. A long ETL reduces the number of slices that can be acquired in a single scan. Also, the longer the ETL, the greater the edge blurring if a short effective TE is chosen and the greater the (artifactual) edge enhancement if a long effective TE is chosen. The blurring/edge enhancement can be minimized by the use of higher receiver bandwidths, which typically result in a shorter "readout" period and thus

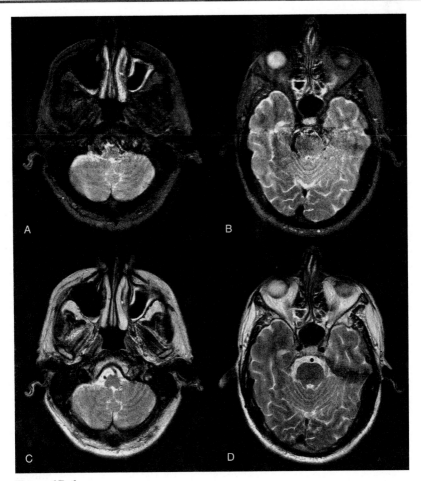

Figure 17–1

reduced time (spacing) between echoes (the critical factor involved). In addition, the multiple 180° RF pulses cause fat to remain high in signal intensity even with long echo times (due to rephasing of stimulated echoes). In this example, the mucosal thickening in the left maxillary sinus is better seen on the conventional spin echo image (Fig. **17–1A**) compared with the FSE image (Fig. **17–1B**), due to the high signal intensity from adjacent fat.

18 Fast Spin Echo (FSE): Reduced Refocusing Angle

Although the reduction in measurement time using multiple phase encoded spin echoes (fast spin echo technique) is very desirable, the use of multiple closely spaced refocusing pulses is associated with higher RF power deposition. Thus a FSE sequence may approach the acceptable limits of specific absorption rate (SAR) relative to patient safety. A common solution to the SAR problem is the use of low refocusing flip angles, which lead to a considerable reduction in SAR at the cost of signal-to-noise ratio (SNR). As indicated in Fig. **18–1,** a refocusing pulse with less than 180° can be considered an insufficient flipping of the dephased fan of transverse magnetizations (2 in Fig. **18–1**). The induced MR signal is diminished, because it is proportional to the part

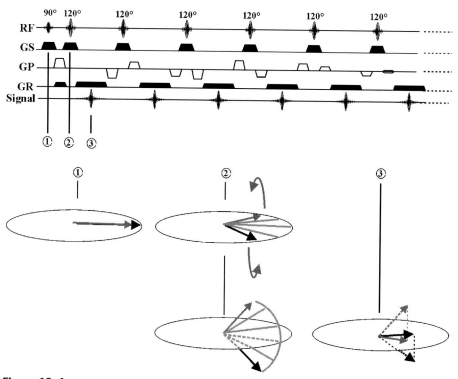

Figure 18–1

of the magnetization projected onto the transverse plane (3 in Fig. **18–1**). Tilting the fan back and forth with a low flip angle refocusing pulse leads to a so-called pseudo–steady state.

Fig. **18–2** presents images acquired with a T2-weighted FSE pulse sequence. Fig. **18–2A** was acquired using 180° refocusing pulses, and **18–2B** was acquired using 120° refocusing pulses. Comparing **A** to **B**, SNR (for white matter, WM) is reduced by 20%, SNR (for CSF) is reduced by 17%, and CNR (WM/CSF) is decreased by 15%. Although the reduction in SNR and CNR, due to use of a flip angle less than 180°, is easily confirmed by region of interest measurements, it is barely perceptible to the average radiologist. The images reveal multiple punctuate areas of increased signal intensity in the cerebral white matter of the centrum semiovale (more prominent anteriorly), consistent with mild chronic small vessel ischemic disease.

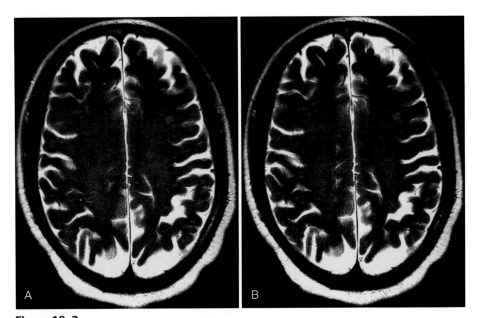

Figure 18–2

The current approaches to decrease power deposition on high field systems (3 T) with methods like TRAPS (transitions between pseudo–steady state) and VFL (variable flip angle imaging) are not to be confused with the simple reduction of the refocusing flip angle in FSE imaging.

19 Reordering: Phase Encoding

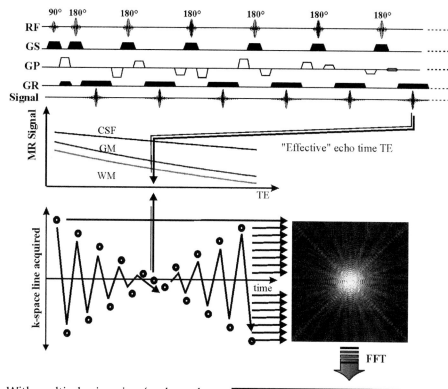

With multiecho imaging (such as that employed with fast spin echo, FSE, technique), where the signal contribution changes during data acquisition, the order in which each k space line is acquired is an important factor in determining image contrast. Given that the low k-space lines contain the information about the coarse structure of the objects within the slice, the echo time at which those k-space lines are acquired is called the "effective" echo time. Although smaller details are presented with a different weighting, the artifacts anticipated with this approach are suppressed due to the higher spatial resolution and the improved contrast in FSE imaging.

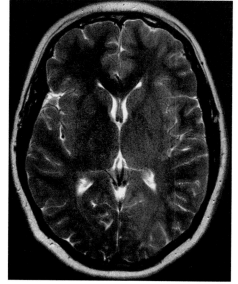

Figure 19–1

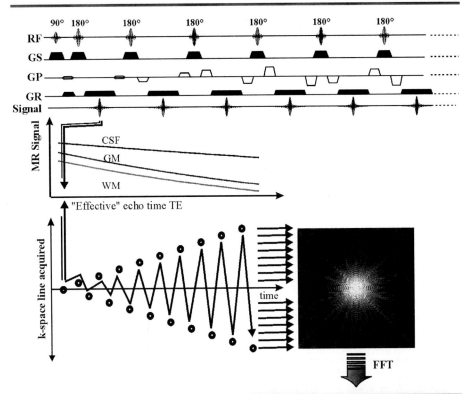

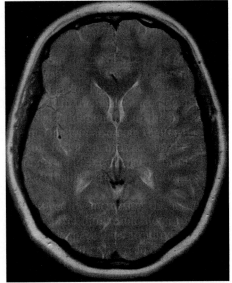

The image shown in Fig. **19–1** was acquired with a long effective TE and thus very heavy T2-weighting. The low k-space lines were acquired in this case at the 10th echo (of the 19 echoes acquired, representing the whole matrix). Alternatively, acquiring the low k-space lines at the very beginning of the echo train, the resulting image is proton density weighted. The image shown in Fig. **19–2** was obtained with an echo train of 19 spin echoes, an echo spacing of 12.1 ms, and with the low k-space lines acquired at the first echo.

Figure 19–2

20 Driven-Equilibrium Fourier Transformation (DEFT)

Driven-equilibrium Fourier transformation (DEFT) is an MRI technique that incorporates the addition of RF pulses at the end of an echo train to drive residual, transverse magnetization back to the longitudinal axis instead of waiting the time required for complete T1 relaxation. This technique is especially useful in situations where the TR for a given sequence would be set higher than what is required for the selected number of slices to wait for tissue relaxation.

Routine, fast spin echo imaging incorporates the initial application of a 90° and 180° RF pulse to form an echo. Additional 180° RF pulses are used to generate subsequent echoes associated with different lines of k space in a given TR period. However, additional time (TR) is often required at the end of the echo train to allow for the recovery of magnetization of tissues with long relaxation times, such as cerebrospinal fluid (CSF) and synovial fluids, resulting in longer acquisition times.

Fig. **20–1A,B** demonstrate the effect TR has on CSF signal intensity in sagittal, fast spin echo acquisitions of the lumbar spine. In Fig. **20–1A,** the TR was decreased to 2000 ms with an acquisition time of about 2 minutes. However, because the time between excitations is not sufficient to allow the longitudinal magnetization of CSF to recover, there is a partial saturation effect and corresponding reduction in the overall signal intensity from CSF. In Fig. **20–1B,** the same sequence was acquired with an increase in TR to 4000 ms, with scan time thus also doubled. The result is higher signal-to-noise ratio (SNR) for CSF due to a reduced saturation effect, but little gain in SNR for other tissues.

DEFT sequences use an additional 180° pulse to refocus the magnetization into one coherent vector in the transverse plane and then a 90° pulse is applied to drive the entire magnetization back to the longitudinal axis. The major benefit is that additional time (TR) is not needed to wait for T1 tissue relaxation, and scan time is reduced due to the decreased TR.

In Fig. **20–1C,D** the same sequence as used in Fig. **20–1A** was acquired in the sagittal and axial plane with the addition of DEFT pulses. The signal contribution from CSF is now similar to that of Fig. **20–1B,** where a higher TR was used. The clear benefit

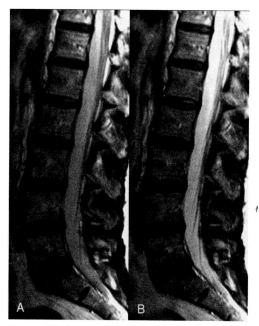

Figure 20–1

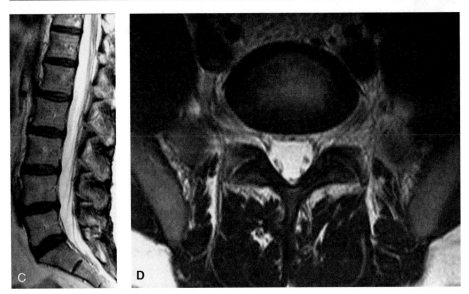

Figure 20–1 (Continued)

in this example is a 50% reduction in acquisition time while maintaining acceptable image quality. The DEFT technique, also called RESTORE, DRIVE, and FR-FSE, continues to be developed and implemented on 2D and 3D spin echo and fast spin echo sequence types with clinical applications in neurologic, orthopedic, and abdominal MRI.

21 Turbo Gradient Spin Echo (TGSE)

The major cause of dephasing during data acquisition is the presence of the readout gradient, GR. Changing the polarity of the gradient creates a gradient echo, with the remaining dephasing due to the tissue specific T2* relaxation time. The combination of gradient echoes with a multiecho fast spin echo approach is called gradient and spin echo (GRASE) or turbo gradient spin echo (TGSE). The upper diagram in Fig. **21–1** is an illustration of a fast spin echo (FSE) sequence. The lower diagram shows a variant of this sequence with three gradient echoes per spin echo envelope, demonstrating that with TGSE more echoes fit into the same echo train length duration, leading to a further reduction in measurement time. Another benefit is the possible larger spacing between 180° RF refocusing pulses, leading to adipose tissue having an intensity similar to that with spin echo (SE) imaging (as opposed to FSE). It is also known that FSE imaging is less sensitive to hemorrhage (specifically deoxyhemoglobin or ferritin) as compared to conventional SE. Because gradient recalled echo (GRE) techniques are known to be highly sensitive to iron in the various blood breakdown products, the combination of gradient echoes with FSE imaging in TGSE increases the sensitivity of the scan for hemorrhage.

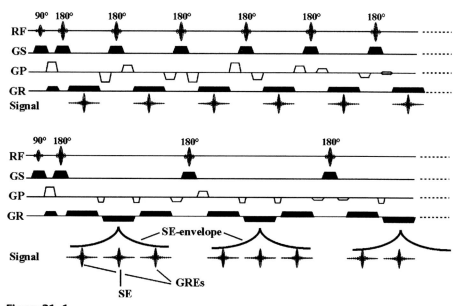

Figure 21–1

Fig. **21–2** presents an exam comparing FSE (Fig. **21–2A,C**) and TGSE (Fig. **21–2B,D**) scans. Measurement times were identical for the two studies. The FSE acquisition was acquired with a 256 × 256 matrix, interpolated to a 512 × 512 displayed matrix. The TGSE sequence was acquired with a true 384 × 512 matrix. The higher intrinsic spatial resolution is possible, within the same scan time, due to acquisition of a greater number of echoes for the same echo train length duration. In this patient with large bilateral subacute subdural hematomas, note the improved detection of iron (with low signal intensity, arrows) within the abnormal extraaxial fluid collections and the lower signal intensity of fat (relative to brain) in the TGSE acquisition.

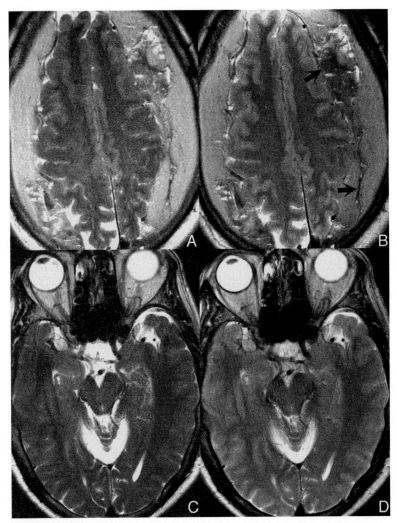

Figure 21–2

22 Half Acquisition Single-Shot Turbo Spin Echo (HASTE)

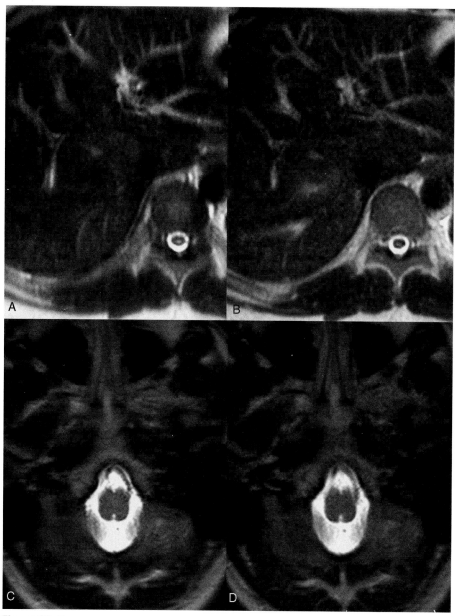

Figure 22–1

Advancements in gradient efficiency and the capability of RF systems on current MR scanners have brought new life to sequences that decrease scan time and minimize the impact of patient motion. One such sequence is HASTE, which stands for half acquisition single-shot turbo spin echo. This approach combines half-Fourier and fast spin echo imaging.

With HASTE, each slice is acquired and often reconstructed before the next slice acquisition has begun. This is accomplished by acquiring an echo train equal to the required number of phase encoding steps for one slice. This differs from normal fast (turbo) spin echo in which phase encoding lines from multiple slices are acquired throughout the examination. The HASTE method also employs a technique known as half-Fourier in which the inherent conjugate symmetry of the raw data is used to synthesize ~50% of the phase encoding steps for each slice. Although there is a corresponding reduction in the signal-to-noise ratio (SNR), spatial resolution is retained. Images with HASTE are usually acquired in 2 seconds or less per slice, making HASTE very good for reducing image quality problems associated with patient motion.

The sampling bandwidth plays an important role in HASTE image quality due to its effect on the spacing of the acquired echoes. If the sampling bandwidth is set too low, resulting in high echo spacing (meaning that there is greater time between each adjacent echo in the train of 128 or so echoes typically used to acquire the image), there can be substantial image blurring (Fig. **22–1A,C**). Selecting a high bandwidth with lower echo spacing (Fig. **22–1B,D**), produces images with slightly lower SNR (see case 96). However, the end result is a much higher diagnostic quality image due to a reduction in image blurring.

HASTE finds clinical applicability, as illustrated, in particular for the upper abdomen and for rapid brain imaging (Fig. **22–2**), with excellent depiction of tissue morphology.

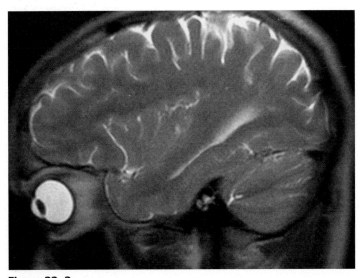

Figure 22–2

23 Inversion Recovery: Part 1

Adipose tissue has a very short T1 relaxation time (~260 ms at 1.5 T), a fact that can be utilized in short tau inversion recovery imaging to eliminate the signal from adipose tissue. As illustrated in Fig. **23–1**, the sequence starts with an inversion pulse. The relatively short inversion time (called short tau), in this case 150 ms, is chosen such that the 90° pulse is applied at a time at which the longitudinal magnetization of adipose tissue is zero and therefore no transverse magnetization is generated. The graph shown in Fig. **23–1** shows the evolution of the longitudinal magnetization following the inversion pulse. The dashed lines in the graph illustrate the theoretical evolution of the longitudinal magnetization with time. For an inversion time, TI, of

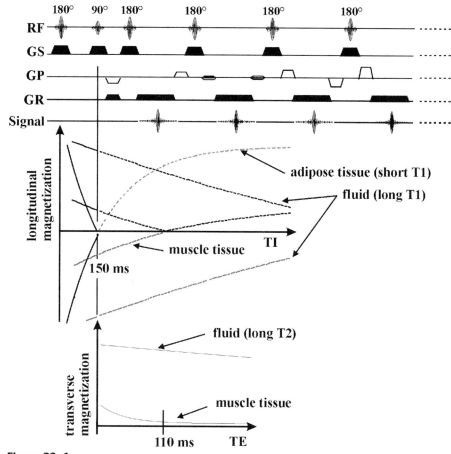

Figure 23–1

150 ms at 1.5 T, the signal of fatty tissue is nulled. In addition, all tissues with short relaxation times will appear darker (for example, muscle). The combination of this technique with T1 shortening contrast agents (e.g., the gadolinium chelates) will increase the effect further. The shortening of T1 due to the administration of contrast media will lead to a further reduction of the available magnetization. The contrast of other tissues relative to fluid-filled cavities can be significantly increased by taking advantage of the long T2 relaxation time and selecting a relatively long echo time as indicated in the lower graph of Fig. **23–1.**

Fig. **23–2** presents a case of a pelvic abscess imaged with a fast spin echo sequence preceded by an inversion pulse with the inversion time chosen to null the signal from fat. The tissue contrast in the image is further enhanced by selecting a long echo time of 110 ms. Fluid-filled regions appear markedly hyperintense. The contrast agent uptake due to inflammatory reaction leads to a further signal reduction, producing an irregular low signal intensity border typical for the image appearance of an abscess (arrow).

For the advanced reader, the inversion time used in spin echo imaging to suppress tissue with a relaxation time of 250 to 260 ms (fat) is between 170 and 180 ms. In fast spin echo imaging, a shorter inversion time has to be selected (~150 ms).

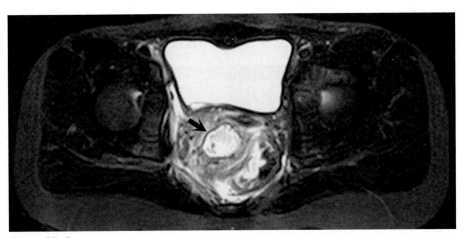

Figure 23–2

24 Inversion Recovery: Part 2

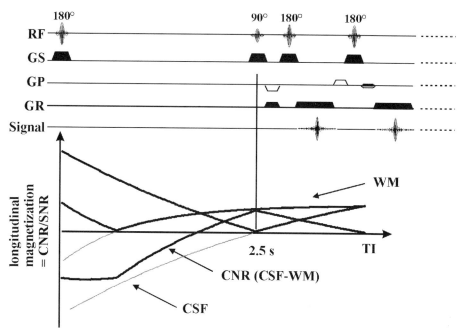

Figure 24–1

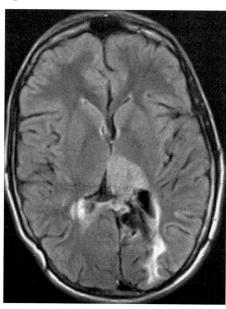

Figure 24–2

With the use of fast spin echo imaging and the resulting savings in scan time, inversion times (TI) on the order of 2.5 seconds (and TRs on the order of 10 seconds) for the suppression of the signal from cerebrospinal fluid (CSF) are possible. In this approach, imaging starts at the time at which the longitudinal magnetization of CSF is zero (Fig. **24–1**). In the resultant image (Fig. **24–2**), CSF will appear black (with little or no signal). In the scan presented, hyperintensity is noted along the surgical tract posteriorly due to gliosis, in this patient with a left thalamic lesion. FLAIR (fluid-attenuated inversion recovery), as this technique is known, is actually a fast spin echo inversion recovery acquisition with a long inversion time.

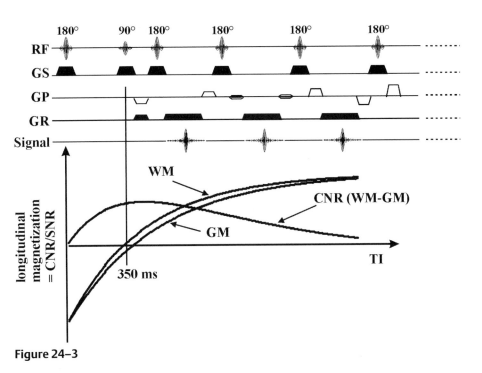

Figure 24–3

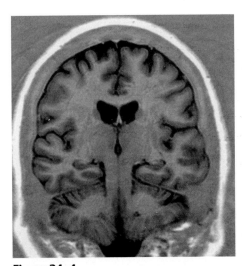

Figure 24–4

"True" inversion recovery acquisitions take into account the "sign" of the longitudinal magnetization (Fig. **24–3**). This is also referred to in the literature as inversion recovery with phase-sensitive reconstruction, as opposed to magnitude reconstruction. In such images, "zero" is displayed as intermediate gray, "negative" signal appears hypointense, and "positive" signal is hyperintense. This technique is especially valuable to study brain maturation, due to the high contrast between gray and white matter (Fig. **24–4**). For phase-sensitive reconstruction, the scale for signal intensity extends from negative to positive (for example –4096 to +4096, with the maximum value vendor specific). For the majority of clinical MR scans acquired today, together with magnitude reconstructed inversion recovery images, the scale extends from 0 to positive.

25 Fluid-Attenuated IR with Fat Saturation (FLAIR FS)

Fluid attenuated inversion recovery with fat saturation (FLAIR FS) takes advantage of the specific (long) relaxation time for pure fluid (cerebrospinal fluid, CSF) and the shift in resonance frequency for adipose tissue to suppress the signal from both. The pulse diagram for this scan technique is illustrated at the top of Fig. **25–1**. The graph below the sequence depicts the temporal evolution, during the course of RF pulses and gradient manipulations, of longitudinal magnetization for adipose tissue, brain tissue and CSF. The inversion time is selected by positioning the 90° RF excitation pulse so that there is no longitudinal magnetization within pure fluid to be converted to transverse magnetization. This is the basic operating principle for FLAIR, resulting in little to no observed signal from CSF. Prior to RF excitation, a frequency selective saturation pulse is issued to saturate any magnetization within adipose tissue. The

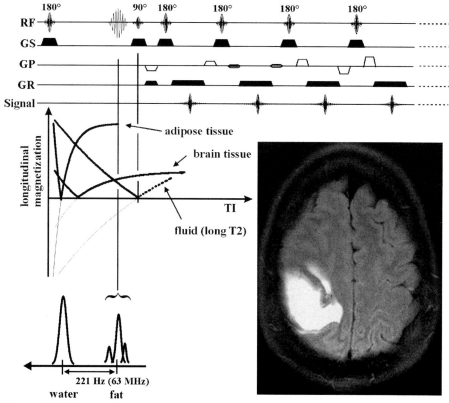

Figure 25–1

resonance frequency for adipose tissue is ~3.5 ppm below that of free water, ~221 Hz on a 1.5 T system. The graph at the bottom of Fig. **25–1** shows the frequency range for carbon-bound hydrogen (fat) and oxygen-bound hydrogen (water) to illustrate the effect of a frequency selective saturation pulse.

Fig. **25–2** presents selected images from the FLAIR scan of a patient who presented acutely with a large intraparenchymal hemorrhage. Mixed blood products are noted within the hematoma. There is substantial surrounding vasogenic edema, with accompanying mass effect upon the right lateral ventricle. Note the low signal intensity of scalp fat, due to the application of fat saturation.

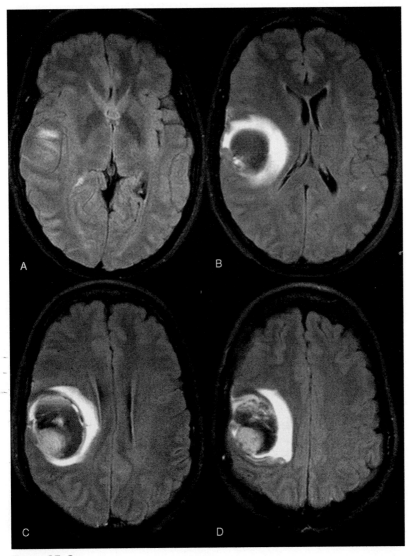

A

B

C

D

Figure 25–2

26 Spoiled Gradient Echo

Cases 26 to 29 demonstrate the evolution from a sequence sampling data during free induction decay to a sequence that also utilizes spin echo contributions. There are several major types of gradient echo sequences, which are discussed in the following pages. This subject is further complicated by the fact that each vendor has its own terminology for the different sequence types.

Fig. **26–1** illustrates a spoiled gradient echo sequence and the signal intensity variation as a function of excitation angle and tissue T1. The use of low flip angle excitation pulses results in only a fraction of the available longitudinal magnetization being tipped into the transverse plane (*1* in Fig. **26–1**). The signal induced in the coil is based on that projection, diminished by the tissue and system specific T2* decay (*2* in Fig. **26–1**). The remaining transverse magnetization is dephased after data acquisition using a "gradient" spoiler (*3* in Fig. **26–1**), or by randomly selecting a different phase for the subsequent RF excitation to avoid any steady-state buildup of transverse magnetization. Unlike spin echo imaging, where all the longitudinal magnetization is converted to transverse magnetization, the longitudinal magnetization is only diminished by the low flip angle excitation. The longitudinal magnetization will further recover, depending on the tissue specific T1-relaxation time (*4* in Fig. **26–1**), until the next low flip angle excitation, which once again creates a transverse magnetization by tipping a fraction of the longitudinal magnetization into the transverse plane. The recovery depends on how far the longitudinal magnetization is away from its fully relaxed state: the further the distance, the faster the recovery. With the next excitation pulse, the longitudinal magnetization is further diminished and after a few

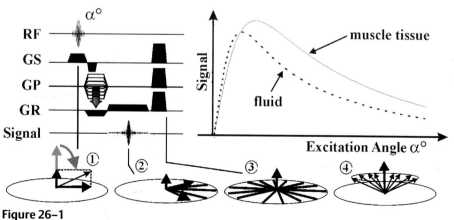

Figure 26–1

measurements, the diminishing action of the low angle excitation will be compensated by the recovery. At this point a steady state for the longitudinal magnetization has been established and the signal for all subsequent Fourier lines will have the same magnitude. Fig. **26–1** also illustrates the change in signal intensity as a function of excitation angle. The maximum signal occurs for an angle called the Ernst angle, which is T1 dependent. This maximum is shifted toward higher excitations angles when using longer TR values. Siemens terms this type of sequence fast low-angle shot (FLASH), General Electric terms it spoiled gradient-recalled acquisition in the steady state (SPGR), and Philips terms it T1 fast field echo (T1-FFE). Sagittal images of the knee using a spoiled gradient echo technique are illustrated in Fig. **26–2**. T1-weighted (short TR and TE, large α), as illustrated (note the depiction of articular cartilage), as well as T2*-weighted (long TR and TE, very small α) contrast can be achieved.

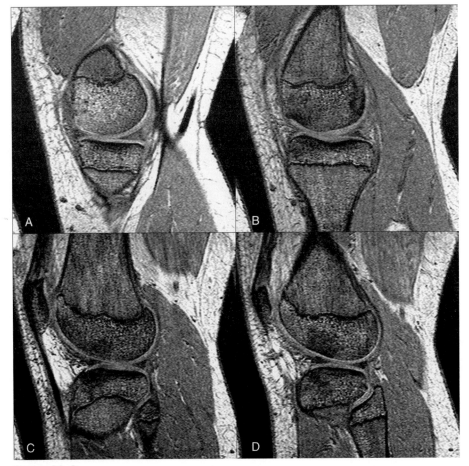

Figure 26–2

27 Refocused (Steady-State) Gradient Echo

Fig. **27–1** illustrates a refocused gradient echo sequence and the signal intensity variation as a function of excitation angle and tissue T1. Excitation, phase encoding, and readout for a refocused gradient echo sequence are identical to that for a spoiled gradient echo sequence (see case 26). Following a low flip angle excitation, only a part of the available longitudinal magnetization is tipped into the transverse plane (*1* in Fig. **27–1**). The induced signal results from the transverse magnetization generated by that excitation and is diminished by the tissue and system specific T2* decay (*2* in Fig. **27–1**), which occurs between excitation and data acquisition. Following data acquisition, however, the remaining transverse magnetization is partially refocused, rather than spoiled (*3* in Fig. **27–1**). The magnetic field gradients used for the purpose of spatial encoding result in a "fanning out" (dephasing) of the transverse magnetization within each voxel. It is common practice to "rewind" the dephasing in the phase encoding direction and call the resulting sequence a refocused gradient echo (GRE). Siemens terms this approach fast imaging with steady precession (FISP), General Electric uses the term gradient-recalled acquisition in the steady state (GRASS), and Philips uses the term fast field echo (FFE).

The rewinding of the transverse magnetization may result in the steady-state transverse magnetization contributing to the signal in addition to the steady-state longitudinal magnetization (*4* in Fig. **27–1**). An additional contribution from residual transverse magnetization is only expected for tissues with long T2* relaxation times. To avoid early dephasing of the transverse magnetization, a short TR value is

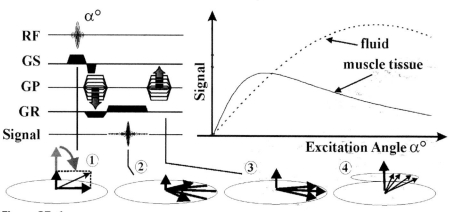

Figure 27–1

necessary, whereas the use of a large flip angle ensures that enough transverse magnetization is generated to contribute in a meaningful way. As illustrated in the plot of signal response as a function of flip angle (Fig. **27–1**), tissue with a long T2* relaxation time, for example synovial fluid (and, in neuroimaging, cerebrospinal fluid), demonstrates an enhanced signal compared with muscle and compared with a spoiled GRE imaging sequence (see Fig. **26–1** in case 26). If the above-mentioned prerequisites are not fulfilled, the signal behavior of a refocused GRE will be identical to that of a spoiled GRE.

Sagittal images of the knee using a refocused GRE scan are shown in Fig. **27–2**. Primarily utilized in musculoskeletal applications, refocused GRE allows for improved delineation of joint fluid (arrow, Fig. **27–2B**). In this instance, the interface between cartilage and the posterior medial meniscus is improved as compared with the spoiled GRE sequence (see Fig. **26–2B** in case 26).

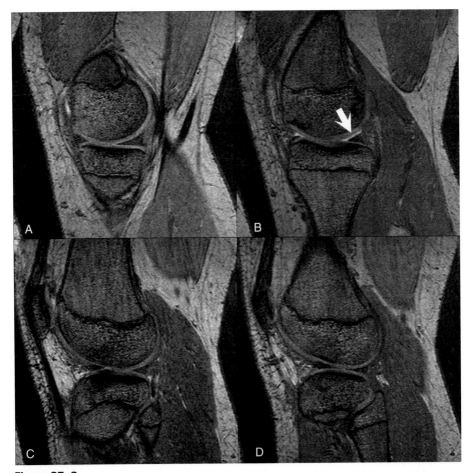

Figure 27–2

28 Dual-Echo Steady State (DESS)

Fig. **28–1** illustrates a double echo steady-state technique, and the signal intensity variation (with this technique) as a function of excitation angle and tissue T1. A further refinement of steady-state gradient echo technique, as illustrated, involves the acquisition of two different echoes during each repetition time (TR). The separation and acquisition of these two echoes are illustrated in Fig. **28–1** and can be described as follows. As noted previously, the signal decay after excitation is called the free induction decay (FID). The FID can be sampled with any gradient echo technique. Any RF excitation pulse also has refocusing capabilities. An echo that is formed using a refocusing RF pulse is called a spin echo (SE). The gradient arrangement for a dual-echo steady-state sequence is such that the first excitation generates a FID, which is sampled, and the refocusing abilities of the next excitation pulse are used to generate a spin echo, which is sampled following the data acquisition of the FID.

The sequence starts with a slice selective low-angle excitation (*1* in Fig. **28–1**), with the FID sampled (*2* in Fig. **28–1**) as for the gradient echo techniques described previously. The remaining transverse magnetization, previously dephased with a phase encoding gradient for the purpose of spatial encoding, is then refocused for that direction. The transverse magnetization is prepared in the direction of slice selection to be refocused in the center of the next excitation pulse, in order to form a spin echo (*3* in Fig. **28–1**). The dephasing mechanism of the slice selection gradient is at this point considered in advance. The frequency encoding gradient is prepared in

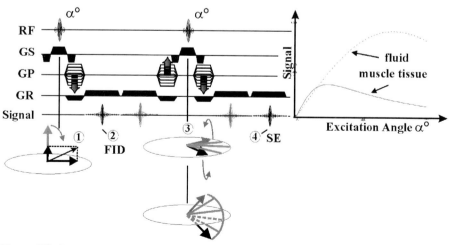

Figure 28–1

such a way that acquisition of the spin echo signal occurs after that of the FID (4 in Fig. **28–1**). Note that the first excitation pulse will produce only a signal in the FID window. In all subsequent excitations, both a FID and a spin echo can be sampled. Note that the effective TE for the spin echo contribution is actually larger than the TR. The FID and SE components are sampled in adjacent windows and combined prior to image reconstruction.

Advantages to this approach, termed double-echo steady-state imaging (DESS, Siemens), include improved signal-to-noise ratio (SNR) (due to acquisition of two echoes that are subsequently combined), stronger T2 contrast, and measurement times comparable to refocused (steady-state) gradient echo technique. Applications include joint imaging, with high signal intensity for fluid, and good delineation of cartilage (Fig. **28–2**).

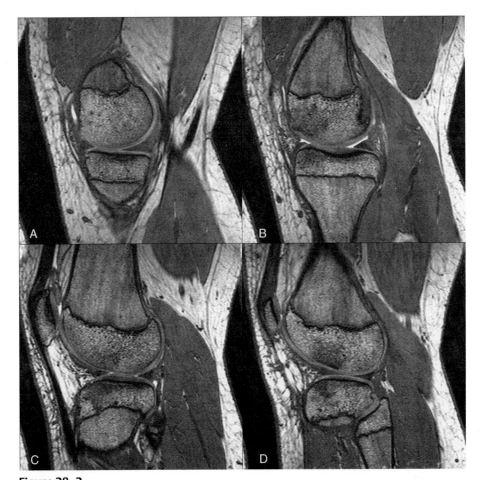

Figure 28–2

29 Balanced Gradient Echo

Fig. **29–1** illustrates a balanced gradient echo sequence and the signal intensity variation (with this approach) as a function of excitation angle and tissue T1. A further refinement of gradient echo technique, as discussed in this case, involves adjusting the free induction decay (FID) component to coincide with the spin echo (SE) component generated by the RF excitation pulse. The first excitation pulse generates the transverse magnetization (*1* in Fig. **29–1**) that will induce the FID signal. The next excitation pulse not only generates transverse magnetization based on the available longitudinal magnetization, but also operates as a RF refocusing pulse for the remaining transverse magnetization of the previous Fourier line measurement (*2* in Fig. **29–1**). The gradient arrangement is adjusted to form (sample) the FID and the SE at the same time (*3* in Fig. **29–1**). Actually, the next excitation pulse operates as a refocusing pulse not only for the remaining magnetization of the FID signal, but also for the remaining magnetization of the SE component. The signal gain is a function of the tissue specific T2-relaxation time. A tissue with a long T2 value appears hyperintense. On inspection of Fig. **29–1,** it can be seen that all gradients are balanced, hence the term *balanced gradient echo*. The transverse magnetizations of all the different echo paths produce a strong signal only if they are pointing in the same direction during the acquisition period; that is, if they are "in phase." Should this not be the case, the resulting signal void is called a destructive interference pattern.

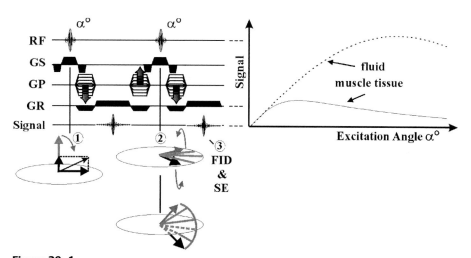

Figure 29–1

Comparing the four different types of gradient echo acquisitions (cases 26–29), there is a progression in signal intensity of fluid, in this instance a small joint effusion, from the first (spoiled) to the last (balanced) technique. It should also be noted that for this particular case, of all four techniques, the balanced gradient echo sequence (Fig. **29–2**) best depicts the bone edema (contusion injury) in both the distal femur and proximal tibia anteriorly (arrows). In regard to terminology, Siemens refers to this approach as true fast imaging with steady precession (trueFISP), General Electric as fast imaging employing steady-state acquisition (FIESTA), and Philips as balanced fast field echo (bFFE).

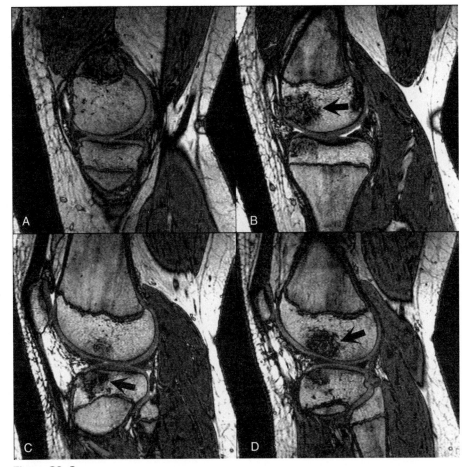

Figure 29–2

30 Steady-State Free-Precession (Balanced GRE)

The examples provided in Fig. **30–1** demonstrate coronal true fast imaging with steady precession (trueFISP) imaging (a balanced gradient echo technique, see case 29) of the upper abdomen (Fig. **30–1A**) without and (Fig. **30–1B**) with fat suppression. Bowel, liver, and, in particular, the vascular system are well defined. It should be noted that the scan time for trueFISP is ~1 second per image.

Fully coherent steady-state free-precession imaging (SSFP) is a gradient echo–based imaging method that has benefited from recent advances in gradient

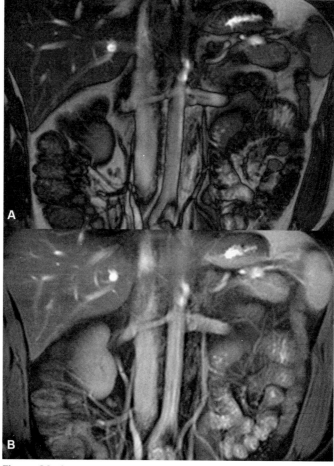

Figure 30–1

hardware and RF amplifier technology. SSFP, also called trueFISP, balanced fast field echo (balanced-FFE), and fast imaging employing steady-state acquisition (FIESTA), is a technique that involves complete rephasing, instead of spoiling, of the transverse magnetization after multiple, rapid excitations. The echo times are kept short through receiver bandwidth settings and advanced hardware, resulting in less sensitivity to artifacts from moving spins such as blood and CSF. This makes SSFP an excellent technique for abdominal and cardiac applications.

The SSFP technique has increased sensitivity to off-resonance effects. Therefore, shimming, similar to that done prior to spectral fat-saturation, is performed before the measurement to improve overall B_0 field homogeneity. Care should also be taken to remove all ferromagnetic objects within the imaging field prior to the examination.

TrueFISP provides the highest signal intensity of all steady-state sequences. Tissue contrast is a function of T1/T2. When acquired with short TR and short TE (as typically implemented), trueFISP provides images that are primarily T2-weighted, with very high signal intensity for all types of fluid (including flowing blood).

Fig. **30–2A** is an axial trueFISP image with fat suppression at the level of the kidneys, with high signal intensity noted from cerebrospinal fluid, fluid within the small bowel (surrounding the pancreatic head), the vascular structures, and urine within the collecting system. Fig. **30–2B** demonstrates the same technique in the sagittal plane, with the anatomy of the right renal hilum well delineated. The gallbladder and hepatic vasculature are depicted, as expected with trueFISP, with high signal intensity.

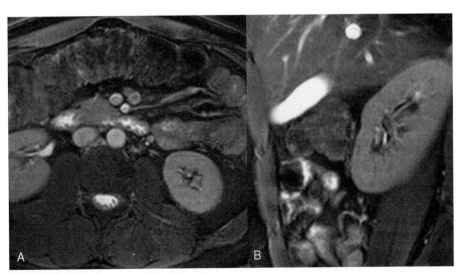

Figure 30–2

31 PSIF: The Backward-Running FISP

It is possible to collect only the spin echo component of the previously described balanced gradient echo. Interestingly, a backward-running FISP generates just the spin echo. The basic sequence loop is illustrated in Fig. **31–1**, indicated between two vertical dashed lines. The excitation pulse for a given acquisition cycle generates transverse magnetization, which is dephased with the gradient arrangement that follows, refocused by the subsequent RF excitation pulse, and read out as spin echo signal. Because the timing is identical to a backward-running FISP, the acronym FISP has been reversed to form PSIF, which has been adopted for this sequence.

Starting with the first excitation pulse, the transverse magnetization dephases in the immediate repetition time interval due to the application of the phase encoding and frequency encoding gradients. No signal is returned during the data acquisition window. In the second cycle, the RF excitation pulse refocuses the dephased magnetization. The signal collected at the echo time is free from T2*-related losses, yielding an image with high T2 contrast. For a PSIF sequence, the echo time is actually longer than the repetition time. The PSIF sequence, although a backward-running FISP, is actually a spin echo sequence. PSIF isolates the spin echo contribution of a balanced gradient echo sequence like trueFISP, FIESTA or bFFE. PSIF is also referred to as a SSFP technique.

Fig. **31–2** demonstrates the difference between PSIF (Fig. **31–2A,C,E**) and constructive interference in a steady state (CISS) (see case 32) (Fig. **31–2B,D,F**) using images at the level of the internal auditory canal. CISS is a phase cycled, balanced gradient echo technique with very low sensitivity to flow. The PSIF signal represents the isolated spin echo of that sequence and is very sensitive to flow. The flow sensitivity

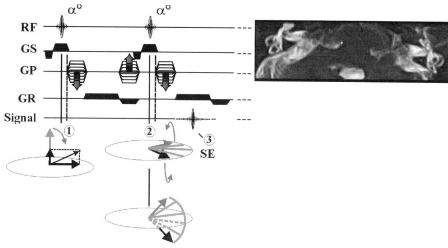

Figure 31–1

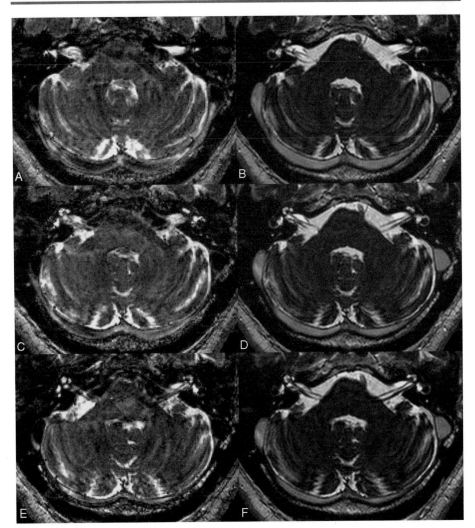

Figure 31 – 2

of PSIF is readily evident in Fig. **31 – 2,** with signal loss in areas of cerebrospinal fluid (CSF) motion, in particular within the prepontine cistern. PSIF, therefore, is not an alternative to display cranial nerves surrounded by CSF, but is a helpful adjunct in cases where the documentation of CSF flow based on the correlated signal void is of diagnostic relevance.

32 Constructive Interference in a Steady State (CISS)

Constructive interference in a steady state (CISS) builds on the fully coherent, steady-state free-precession technique (SSFP) (see case 30), resulting in a high-resolution, 3D imaging sequence with good fluid sensitivity and strong T2 (water) weighting.

In the absence of a perfectly homogeneous magnetic field, dark band artifacts can occur in routine SSFP images. To increase homogeneity and reduce the occurrence of such artifacts, the field is shimmed. However, in areas of the head such as the internal auditory canals, susceptibility differences between air and tissue lead to an increase in magnetic field inhomogeneity, making banding artifacts difficult to minimize. Alterations in the phase of SSFP acquisitions can shift the position of these artifacts, and are employed in CISS.

The CISS sequence works by collecting two 3D SSFP data sets with slight differences in phase causing shifts in the position of dark band artifacts between data sets. Prior to reconstruction, a complex addition of the two raw data sets is done, similar to a maximum intensity projection, filling areas where dark bands would appear and leading to a square root of two increase in the signal-to-noise ratio (SNR). The Fourier transform of the new data set results in an image largely free of dark band artifacts.

Images are presented from a patient with a very small left-sided intracanalicular acoustic schwannoma. Axial fast spin echo T2-weighted (Fig. **32–1A**), contrast enhanced, spin echo T1-weighted (Fig. **32–1B**), and CISS (Fig. **32–1C**) sequences were acquired through the internal auditory canals. The lesion is difficult to detect on the fast spin echo T2-weighted image. However, the CISS sequence displays well the focal enlargement of the nerve (arrow, Fig. **32–1C**) within the canal, and thus enables detection of this small tumor. Indeed the lesion was visualized on two adjacent slices from the CISS scan. Due to enhancement, the lesion is also well visualized on the T1-weighted postcontrast spin echo scan (arrow, Fig. **32–1B**).

The heavily T2-weighted, 3D CISS sequence is often acquired with high spatial resolution and submillimeter partitions, offering detailed delineation of small structures of the inner ear and cerebellopontine angle. 3D CISS scans can be processed using maximum intensity and surface rendering algorithms, with the result being, when acquired with an isotropic voxel, high-quality 3D reconstructions of the cochlea, vestibule, and semicircular canals (Fig. **32–1D**).

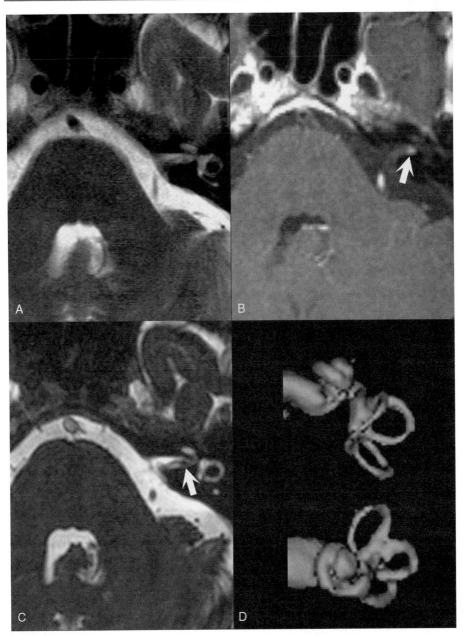

Figure 32 – 1

33 TurboFLASH, FSPGR, TFE

In the case of fast gradient echo imaging sequences with low-angle excitation and very short TR and TE values, it is possible to achieve strong T1-weighting using an inversion recovery–based approach. Instead of applying an inversion pulse prior to the acquisition of each Fourier line (which would imply a very long measurement time), the inversion pulse is applied once at the beginning of the acquisition. The preparation of the magnetization can also be performed with a "saturation recovery" pulse (SR), which is a 90° RF pulse, saturating all tissues prior to the start of the imaging sequence. As illustrated in Fig. **33 – 1**, the magnetization recovers immediately following the preparing pulse. For the duration of the acquisition time, the relaxation curve is influenced by the low-angle excitation and the repetition time (TR). This technique is used preferentially in perfusion imaging. The time between the preparation pulse and the time the center of k space is acquired is called the inversion time (TI). Such a technique provides excellent visualization of the first pass of a contrast agent through the cardiac chambers followed by contrast uptake in normal myocardium. Sequence acronyms for this technique include FSPGR—fast spoiled gradient acquisition in the

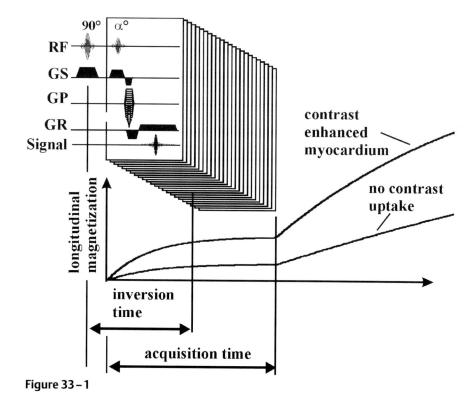

Figure 33 – 1

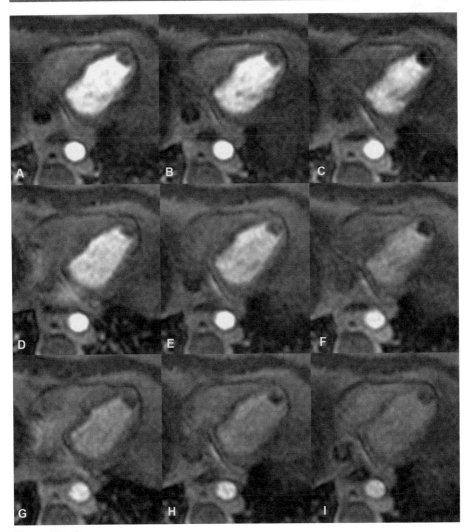

Figure 33–2

steady state (General Electric), TFE – turbo field echo (Philips), and turboFLASH – turbo fast low angle shot (Siemens).

Fig. **33–2A–I** presents images during the first pass of a contrast bolus through the left ventricle employing a turboFLASH sequence (one image per heart beat). A nonenhancing mass-like lesion (corresponding to thrombus), with associated apical thinning, is visible at the apex of the left ventricle in this patient with a history of prior myocardial infarction. It should also be noted that, although this is a common application of contrast media in clinical practice, no agent is strictly approved for this use by the Food and Drug Administration (FDA) and thus the use is off-label.

34 Faster and Stronger Gradients: Part 1

Fig. **34 – 1A** is an illustration of the consequences of a stronger and faster gradient system on the imaging capabilities of a gradient echo sequence. The frequency range for the excited slice is usually untouched, dictating the amplitude for the slice select gradient (GS). The same situation applies to the selected bandwidth per pixel, dictating

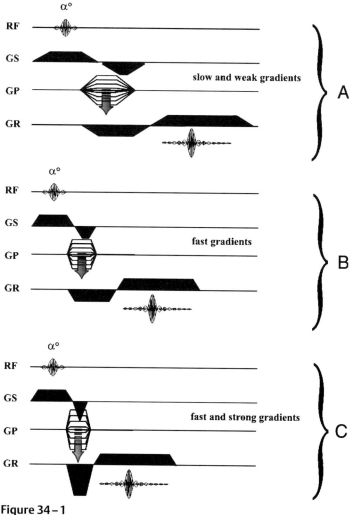

Figure 34 – 1

the amplitude for the readout gradient (GR) during readout. The most important part, therefore, is how fast the gradients can achieve their nominal value, so that the excitation can be activated or the data sampled. The faster the gradient (Fig. **34–1B**), the shorter the time between tasks, the shorter the echo time (that can be achieved), the shorter the slice loop, and the shorter the repetition time (that can be achieved). A shorter echo time or echo spacing in fast spin echo imaging also leads to an improved signal contribution to the image. A stronger gradient (Fig. **34–1C**) also allows some of the preparation pulses to become shorter, permitting further shortening of TE and TR. Stronger gradients also allow the same bandwidth for a smaller field of view, enabling high-resolution imaging if permitted by the signal-to-noise ratio. A stronger gradient system can also be beneficial for some specific applications, for example diffusion-weighted imaging.

Fig. **34–2** is a comparison, in a normal volunteer, using a trueFISP or balanced gradient echo imaging application. Fig. **34–2A** has been acquired with "strong" gradients, whereas Fig. **34–2B** has been acquired with "weak" gradients. As a consequence, the echo time increased from 2.15 ms (Fig. **34–2A**) to 2.59 ms (Fig. **34–2B**). Because the echo time also dictates the minimum repetition time, the latter increased from 4.3 ms to 5.18 ms. Although these appear to be minor changes, it has to be kept in mind that balanced gradient echo imaging relies on a short TR to gain additional signal for tissues with long T2 relaxation times. In the example presented, the gain in repetition time is only 0.88 ms, yet the signal gain for tissues with long T2 relaxation time is quite evident, with cerebrospinal fluid of substantially higher signal intensity in Fig. **34–2A** (arrow).

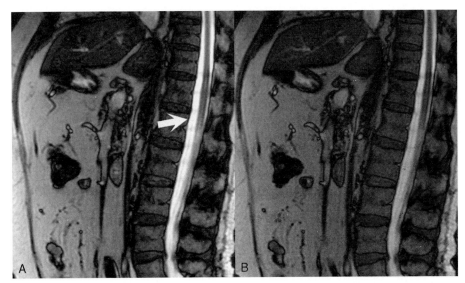

Figure 34–2

35 Faster and Stronger Gradients: Part 2

Fig. **35–1** illustrates the effect of a faster and stronger gradient system on fast spin echo imaging. The benefits applicable to imaging with a single echo (previously discussed) also translate into significant improvements when using multi-echo methods such as fast spin echo. The most important factor here is "faster" gradients, that is, minimizing the time for the gradients to reach their nominal value. Once they have achieved their nominal value, the excitation or refocusing pulse can be issued, or data sampling can be initiated. The "strength" of the gradient has less, but some, impact on the speed of acquisition. Specifically, for the GR preparation pulse, only the time-amplitude integral is of importance (maintaining this value, whether using stronger or weaker gradients). Increasing the amplitude of that pulse allows the application of a shorter duration while achieving the same preparatory dephasing of the transverse magnetization. The same can be done for the phase encoding gradient with a shorter gradient duration possible with use of higher gradient amplitude.

As illustrated in Fig. **35–1,** a faster and stronger gradient system permits the echo spacing to be shorter in multi-echo imaging. This makes possible sampling of more echoes within the same time (which could be used to shorten scan time), or alternatively allows more slices to be acquired for the same given repetition time.

Fig. **35–2** shows a comparison of T2-weighted fast spin echo acquisitions with different gradient settings in a normal patient. Fig. **35–2A** was acquired using a "strong" gradient setting, whereas Fig. **35–2B** was acquired using a "weak" gradient setting. There is no difference in image quality other than a slight inadvertent change

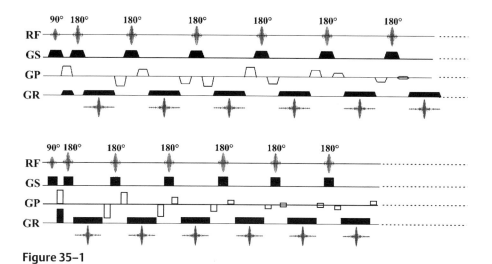

Figure 35–1

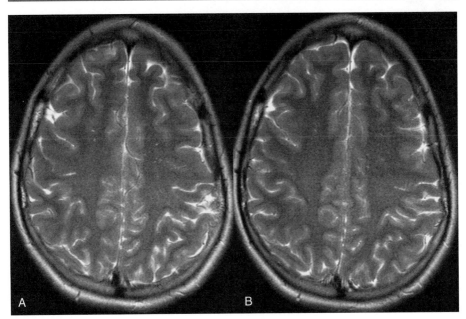

Figure 35–2

in slice position due to patient movement. Changing gradient strength from "strong" to "weak" increased echo spacing from 12.1 ms to 13.6 ms. This dictates an increase in echo train length (ETL) from 230 ms to 258 ms for 19 echoes. With the change in ETL, the slice-loop time also increased from 239 ms to 268 ms. As a consequence, the number of slices had to be decreased from 22 to 19 for the same given TR.

36 Multislice Imaging and Concatenations

The time needed to excite and spatially encode one slice is called the slice-loop time (Fig. **36–1**). The time between the excitation pulses for the same slice is the repetition time and is a major contrast-dictating parameter. On completion of encoding of a given slice, there is time prior to the next excitation pulse to excite and encode other slices. For this approach, called multislice imaging, the maximum number of slices is given by the repetition time divided by the slice-loop time. If more slices are needed than fit into the requested TR, the acquisition can be "concatenated" (Fig. **36–2**).

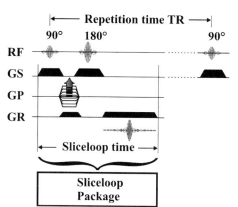

Figure 36–1

In other words, the number of slices is evenly split into the desired number of concatenations. In doing so the TR remains unchanged. The measurement time is proportional to the number of concatenations. For fast spin echo imaging, the slice-loop time includes the slice-selective excitation and the echo train length (ETL). As is evident from Fig. **36–2**, selecting concatenations may waste measurement time (causing the scan to be unnecessarily long). Concatenations should be selected, if T1-weighting (and the specified short TR) is absolutely essential.

The strength of a gradient system is given by its maximum amplitude and the rise time required to achieve that amplitude. Faster ramping (higher performance gradients) shortens the time for ramping up and down the encoding gradients. Because the latter has to be performed multiple times in a multi-echo sequence, the space between echoes is shorter and the whole ETL becomes shorter. The slice-loop

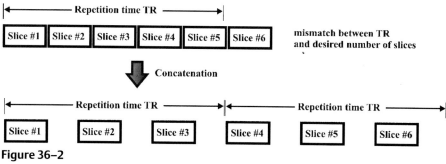

Figure 36–2

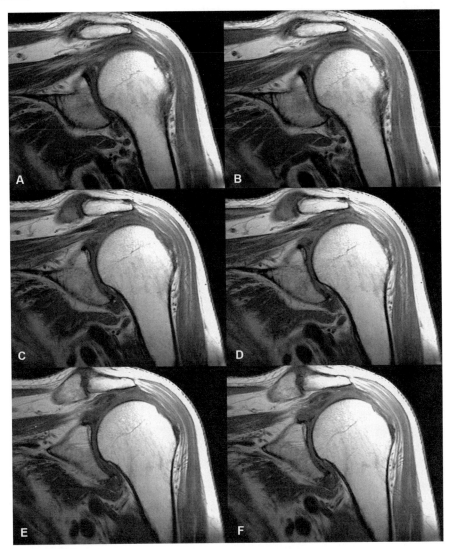

Figure 36–3

time is a function of ETL, and it also decreases. In that case more slices fit into one TR interval and concatenations may be avoided.

Fig. **36–3A–F** presents images of a patient with a full-thickness partial width tear of the supraspinatus tendon. The left column of images was acquired with a repetition time of 637 ms and two concatenations. The images in the right column were acquired with a repetition time of 1280 ms (and only one concatenation). Scan times were identical. The images in the right column have better proton density weighting, due to the longer TR. The SNR in tendon and skeletal muscle is also increased by ~15%.

37 3D Imaging: Basic Principles

A low signal intensity extraaxial lesion (black arrow) is noted on a 2D T2-weighted scan with a 5-mm slice thickness (Fig. **37–1A**). The lesion is seen on multiple contiguous 1-mm T1-weighted scans (Fig. **37–1B**) from a 3D acquisition. There is heterogeneous contrast enhancement (white arrow), with the lesion, which lies in the left frontal region along the convexity, corresponding to a small meningioma. Fig. **37–1C,D** employs the same scan techniques, respectively, as Fig. **37–1A,B**, with the 1-mm contiguous 3D sections (Fig. **37–1D**) providing detailed depiction of the sylvian fissure.

There are two main approaches to acquiring MR images: 2D and 3D. In most situations, a slice is selectively excited by use of a gradient magnetic field (slice-select gradient) and then encoded in two dimensions (phase encoding and readout). This type of technique is known as two-dimensional Fourier transform (2D-FT). The images in Fig. **37–1A,C** are examples of such an acquisition. The second way to acquire the data is to excite an entire volume, or slab, rather than a single slice. To produce slices from the slab, additional phase encodings are applied along the slice direction. This technique is known as 3D-FT (commonly referred to as a volume acquisition). The images in Fig. **37–1B,D** were acquired in a 3D fashion using a gradient echo pulse sequence known as MP-RAGE (see case 38).

The number of slices, or partitions, desired determines the number of phase encoding steps required along the slice direction of the slab in a 3D acquisition. As an example, if one desires 20 slices, then 20 phase encodings are performed along the slice direction. If the total size of the slab is 100 mm, then those slice encodings produce 20 slices with a slice thickness of 5 mm. If the number of slices desired is increased to 40, and the total slab size remains the same, the result would be 40 slices with a slice thickness of 2.5 mm. In any 3D sequence (other than MP-RAGE, which is performed in a quite different way from conventional 3D imaging), the number of slice encodings applied directly affects scan time. In the previous example, the 40-slice data set would require twice the number of slice encodings as the 20-slice data set. As such, the scan time of the 40-slice data set would be twice that of the 20-slice data set.

There are several benefits to a 3D acquisition. Slices are produced with no gap or spacing between them. Because the slices are encoded, rather than excited as in a 2D acquisition, there is no crosstalk between slices, as may be seen in a 2D acquisition (which leads to a loss of SNR and changes in image contrast in 2D). Additionally, 3D acquisitions inherently have higher SNR because a slab is excited rather than a single, thin slice. This makes 3D particularly attractive for use at low field strengths. Lastly, if one were to acquire the data set using an isotropic voxel (voxel dimensions equal in all three dimensions), or simply a small voxel with near equal dimensions in all three axes, the data set may be reformatted with high resolution in any plane.

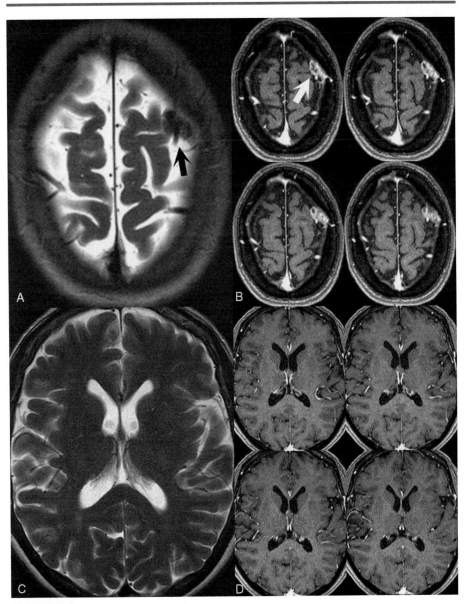

Figure 37–1

38 MP-RAGE (3D TurboFLASH)

The challenge of extending turboFLASH from 2D acquisition to 3D acquisition is due to the fact that the effect of an inversion pulse applied at the very beginning of the acquisition is lost during the acquisition. This is due to the high number of excitation pulses and the relatively long measurement time associated with 3D acquisitions. This may be overcome by repeating the inversion pulse during the measurement. Three-dimensional image acquisition requires a repetition of all phase encoding steps in the slab (partition) direction for every phase encoding step within the imaging plane. The inversion pulse is placed prior to the partition encoding loop. Within the partition encoding loop (GS(P)), the signal is changing due to recovery of the longitudinal magnetization (Fig. **38–1**). However, the signal contribution along the Fourier lines of phase encoding within the imaging plane is constant (GP(P)). Consequently, the blurring artifact observed in turboFLASH imaging is visible only for images reconstructed in the partition encoding direction. This technique is called magnetization-prepared rapid gradient echo (MP-RAGE) (Fig. **38–1**).

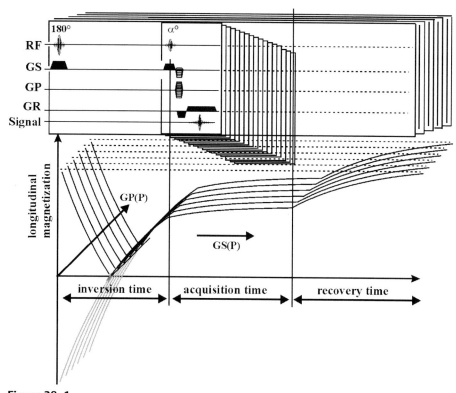

Figure 38–1

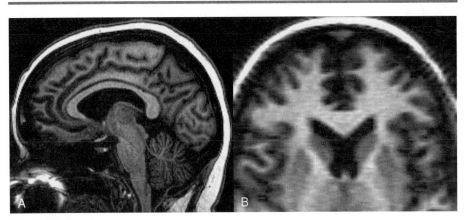

Figure 38–2

There are several advantages to using MP-RAGE for T1-weighted imaging. Unlike multislice 2D imaging, the partition encoding used in 3D acquisitions, such as in MP-RAGE, allows for continuous coverage with thin slices in a reasonable measurement time (~6 minutes). Inversion of the magnetization allows better control over T1-weighting, permitting greater T1 contrast compared with SE imaging. Fig. **38–2** presents sagittal (Fig. **38–2A**) and axial (Fig. **38–2B**) images of a normal volunteer acquired with an MP-RAGE sequence; the contrast between gray and white matter is particularly noteworthy. Note also the accentuated blurring in Fig. **38–2B,** the reformatted acquisition, as opposed to that in Fig. **38–2A,** the primary plane. The susceptibility artifact due to metal within the oral cavity (Fig. **38–2A**) is a reminder that MP-RAGE is a gradient echo technique. Fig. **38–3** shows a sagittal, postcontrast acquisition of a patient with a dermoid cyst (note the fat/fluid level). Although very attractive, MP-RAGE has not replaced T1-weighted spin echo imaging for postcontrast scans. There have been reports of poor visualization of enhancing lesions with MP-RAGE. This may be attributed to the fact that following contrast agent administration, a lesion may appear isointense with adjacent normal, but high signal intensity, white matter.

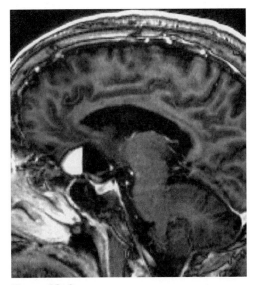

Figure 38–3

39 Echo Planar Imaging

Echo planar imaging (EPI) is one of the fastest techniques for acquiring MRI data. This method incorporates rapid changes in readout gradient polarity and amplitude to refocus the signal of a single spin excitation, producing the required echoes for an entire image. The acquisition time for one slice is one TR period, which lasts as little as 100 ms, and the process is repeated for the number of slices desired.

Echo planar imaging techniques are defined by the spin preparation method used. Gradient echo (GRE-EPI) consists of a single RF excitation creating a free induction decay (FID)-based image. A dual RF pulse train generates an RF echo, which is the basis for spin echo (SE-EPI) images. Inversion pulses (IR-EPI) can also be applied to obtain fluid-attenuated inversion recovery (FLAIR)-like echo planar images.

Collecting enough information for a complete slice in one sampling period requires that the MR gradient hardware be capable of reaching a high level of gradient change (peak amplitude) in a short period of time (rise time). The peak amplitude divided by the rise time is a gradient performance measurement known as the slew rate. Higher slew rates allow EPI information to be collected in shorter time intervals, leading to higher quality images with less distortion caused by increased echo spacing.

Spectral fat saturation is used to reduce the presence of chemical shift artifact induced by the extreme field sensitivity of EPI scans and the systematic errors between the odd and even echoes generated during the readout portion of the sequence. This artifact, often referred to as N/2 or Nyquist ghosting, would otherwise obscure the water image.

Axial images are presented from a patient with an anaplastic astrocytoma. Due to the size of the tumor and associated edema, there is substantial mass effect upon the brainstem. Fast spin echo T2 (Fig. **39–1A**), FLAIR (Fig. **39–1C**), and spin echo T1-weighted postcontrast (Fig. **39–1E**) images are compared with EPI acquisitions (Fig. **39–1B,D,F**) at the same slice position with similar weightings. In each case, the EPI examples showed a reduction in scan time of 50% or greater while maintaining overall image contrast. Another major difference is that the spin echo scans are multislice in technique (with motion at any time during the scan acquisition affecting all slices), whereas the EPI images are single slice and thus very robust in regard to patient motion. Note the ghosting (arrow) due to inadvertent patient motion on the postcontrast T1-weighted spin echo scan (Fig. **39–1E**), which is absent on the corresponding EPI scan (Fig. **39–1F**). EPI finds clinical applicability in diffusion, perfusion, and functional neurologic imaging, and, due to its single slice acquisition method, is an excellent tool for reducing artifacts associated with patient motion.

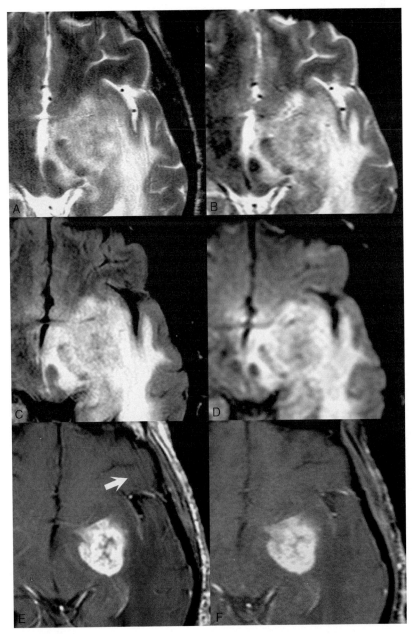

Figure 39–1

40 Flow Effects: Fast and Slow Flow

Fig. **40–1** presents images from two separate scans in the same patient, varying only the number of slices acquired. In Fig. **40–1A**, images were acquired on both sides of the slice illustrated, whereas in Fig. **40–1B** fewer slices were acquired. More specifically, the scan illustrated in Fig. **40–1B** is that from the outermost slice. Thus despite identical scan technique in terms of T1 weighting, Fig. **40–1B** illustrates inflow effects (flow related enhancement) in the cortical veins (arrows) draining into the sagittal sinus, which are absent in Fig. **40–1A.**

Flow is an intrinsic contrast mechanism in MR, analogous to some degree to T1, T2, and proton density. The signal intensity of flow depends on the pulse sequence selected, the velocity, and the presence or absence of turbulence, as well as the method in which the slice or volume of data are acquired. A spin echo pulse sequence consists of a 90° RF pulse followed by a 180° pulse. Both pulses are slice selective and thus any tissue or substance within the slice that receives both pulses can produce an MR signal (given the proper TR and TE). Blood is no exception. If the blood flowing into the slice has not been presaturated by an RF pulse outside the imaging volume, and it is flow-

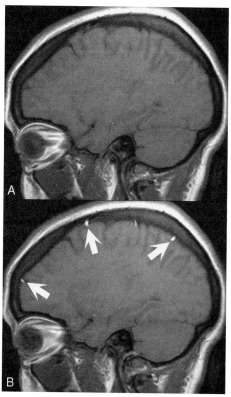

Figure 40–1

ing slowly enough to receive both the 90° and 180° pulse, then it can have high signal intensity (flow-related enhancement). This is well demonstrated by the high signal intensity seen in the cortical veins in Fig. **40–1B**. It should also be noted that flow-related enhancement is more prevalent when blood flows perpendicular to the slice. On the other hand, if the blood is flowing fairly rapidly so that it does not receive both RF pulses, or if it has become saturated as it flows through a multislice data set or volume, then it will have little (Fig. **40–1A**) to no signal intensity, the latter being a flow "void."

Fig. **40–2** is from a pediatric patient with stenosis (obstruction) of the cerebral aqueduct, resulting in long-standing enlargement of the third and lateral ventricles. Fig. **40–2A** and Fig. **40–2B** are sagittal T1-weighted spin echo scans, and Fig. **40–2C** an axial T2-weighted fast spin echo scan. Flow (signal) voids are noted in the basilar artery (arrow, Fig. **40–2A**), cavernous carotid artery (arrow, Fig. **40–2B**), and in the superior sagittal sinus and draining cortical veins (arrows, Fig. **40–2C**).

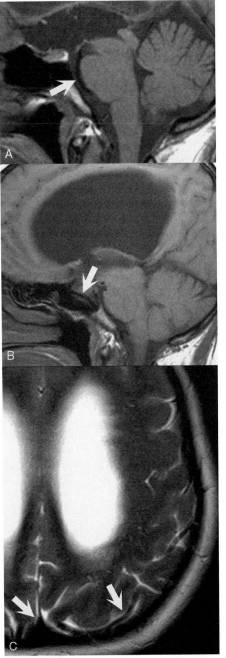

Figure 40–2

As illustrated, flowing blood (arterial or venous) can produce either a signal void or high signal depending on (in particular) flow velocity, vessel orientation relative to the slice, and, most importantly, the pulse sequence selected. In general, spin echo sequences depict flowing blood as a signal void (with some exceptions as noted). Vascular imaging using spin echo based scans is sometimes referred to as "black blood" or "dark blood" technique. Gradient echo sequences depict flowing blood as high signal, particularly when acquired in a single-slice fashion [or as a single "slab" as in 3D time-of-flight magnetic resonance angiography (TOF MRA)] to take advantage of flow-related enhancement. Images of blood flow acquired with gradient echo sequences may be referred to as "bright blood" technique and are the basis for TOF MRA.

41   2D Time-of-Flight MRA

Two-dimensional time-of-flight (2D TOF) technique has been used for many years to acquire images of blood flow in the carotid arteries. The basic pulse sequence is a 2D spoiled gradient echo [fast low-angle shot (FLASH)] in which axial slices are acquired in a sequential fashion. In a sequential acquisition, a single slice is completely acquired before the next. A fairly short repetition time (TR) is used together with a relatively high flip angle. This results in reduced signal from background (stationary) tissue, as there is insufficient time for recovery of longitudinal magnetization (T1 relaxation). In such a situation, the background tissue is said to be "saturated." On the other hand, protons moving into the slice (flow) have full longitudinal magnetization, as they have yet to be exposed to an RF pulse. The net result is that blood flowing into the slice has high signal intensity. The high signal resulting from the inflow of unsaturated blood protons is referred to as "flow-related enhancement" and is the basic contrast mechanism in a TOF acquisition. To eliminate the signal from the jugular veins, an additional RF pulse is applied superior to the axial slice. This presaturation pulse (see case 101) moves together with the axial slice as each subsequent slice is acquired. Blood flowing in the craniocaudal direction (in the jugular veins) is thus saturated as it flows into the imaging slice and produces no MR signal.

The axial images from a 2D TOF acquisition (sometimes referred to as the "source images") in a patient with a severe stenosis just distal to the origin of the left internal carotid artery are shown in Fig. **41–1A**. To view the images in a more convenient and familiar fashion, the images are "stacked" and a postprocessing technique known as maximum intensity projection (MIP) employed to produce "angiographic-like" projection images (Fig. **41–1B**). It is important to remember that the MIP images are not an "angiogram" but rather a projection produced from the axial data set. Any tissue or substance with a short T1-relaxation time (such as fat or methemoglobin), depending on the exact scan technique used, may be hyperintense on the axial data set, and thus on MIP images obscure blood flow or even potentially be confused for flow. One will also notice two areas of signal misregistration (arrows) in Fig. **41–1B**. This is due to patient motion during or between slice acquisitions in the sequential 2D scan. When interpreting scans, it is important to review both the MIP and source images. The latter provide a means of assessing surrounding tissues and anatomy, and often make easier identification of artifacts due to motion, signal loss (metal clips), and the presence of fat or methemoglobin.

It is well known that complex flow, such as that seen with turbulence, is not easily compensated for and can result in artifactual signal loss. Complex flow patterns can, and often do, result in an exaggeration of MR signal loss in the area of a stenotic lesion, and thus an overestimation of the degree of stenosis. Although the slice thickness of 2D TOF sequences is usually less than 2.0 mm, 3D acquisitions can be used to produce images with thinner slices, which together with the use of shorter TEs (as generally employed in 3D TOF MRA), greatly reduces the artifactual signal loss. 3D TOF techniques also do not demonstrate the misregistration artifact previously described.

Although 2D TOF does overestimate the degree of stenosis, it has been shown to be an effective screening technique for carotid artery disease. The addition of 3D TOF

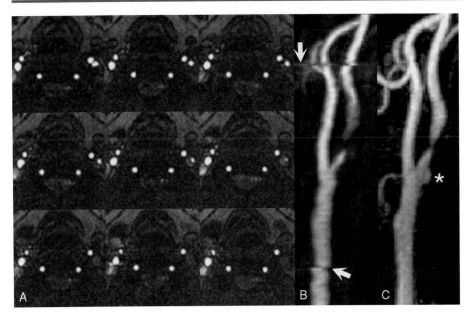

Figure 41–1

sequences aids in reducing artifactual signal loss due to complex flow patterns. However, contrast-enhanced MRA (CE-MRA), because of decreased scan time (minimizing the effects of patient motion) and reduced sensitivity to complex flow patterns, has replaced 2D TOF in most applications. The MIP image in Fig. **41–1C** is from a 3D CE-MRA acquisition. It demonstrates less artifactual signal loss in the area of stenosis, and also permits identification of an ulcerated plaque (*) just proximal to the stenosis.

42 3D Time-of-Flight MRA

A 6-mm saccular aneurysm is seen arising from the right side of the anterior communicating artery (arrow, Fig. **42–1C**) on the maximum intensity projection (MIP) image of the circle of Willis. On the T2-weighted fast spin echo sequence, the aneurysm is seen as a flow void (arrow, Fig. **42–1A**). The aneurysm is also well seen on the source images from the 3D time-of-flight MRA scan (Fig. **42–1B**).

Flow is an intrinsic contrast mechanism that can be imaged with MRI in several ways. Spin echo (SE) sequences utilize a 90° RF pulse followed by a 180° RF pulse to produce an echo (the observed signal). In standard imaging sequences, both the 90° and 180° pulses are slice selective. In typical vessels with normal flow velocities, blood is not in the slice to receive both RF pulses, and thus flow is seen as a signal void (Fig. **42–1A**). Gradient echo (GRE) sequences utilize only a single RF excitation pulse and the echo is formed by a gradient magnetic field reversal only. In this situation, blood that flows into the slice is hyperintense. This is particularly true when a short TE is used.

Time-of-flight (TOF) MRA uses GRE sequences to depict flowing blood as bright signal. TOF sequences can be acquired in either a 2D (slice-by-slice) or 3D (volume excitation) fashion. A 3D sequence allows for thinner slices (higher spatial resolution). Small voxel size and a short TE are important for producing MRA scans with minimal signal loss due to flow artifacts. Additionally, 3D acquisitions can produce images with very high signal-to-noise ratio (SNR) despite the use of very thin slices. High SNR and spatial resolution are critical when imaging flow within the intracranial vasculature. In routine clinical practice today, the major use of 3D TOF MRA is for imaging of the circle of Willis (for aneurysms and vascular stenoses/occlusion).

In an MRA sequence, the slices, or in this case the volume, is acquired with a fairly short TR. The background tissue becomes saturated and does not yield a very strong MR signal. Blood, on the other hand, when flowing at normal velocities, flows through the slice or volume and is not given time to become saturated. As fresh, unsaturated, blood continues to flow into the slice or volume, it produces a strong MR signal. This is known as flow related enhancement.

The source images acquired during the 3D acquisition (Fig. **42–1B**) are then processed using one of several techniques, the most common today being MIP. Surface or volume rendering is also possible on many MR systems, and represents an alternative postprocessing technique. Using MIP, multiple projections, or views, are produced. Fig. **42–1C** is one such projection. It is important to realize that the MIP projections are not the actual acquired images and may not always clearly demonstrate pathology. As such, the source images should be reviewed as well.

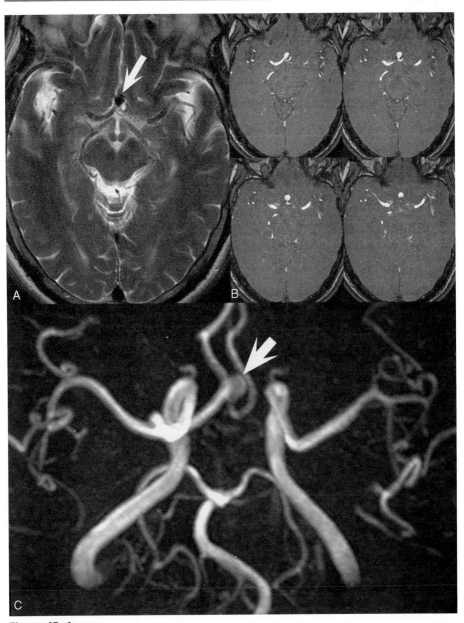

Figure 42–1

43 Flip Angle and MT in 3D Time-of-Flight MRA

Three-dimensional time-of-flight (3D TOF) magnetic resonance angiography (MRA) continues to be the dominant MR technique for imaging the intracranial arterial vasculature. As discussed in case 42, the contrast between flow and stationary tissue relies on a balance of saturation between the background and flowing blood (with preferential saturation of the former). This is especially difficult to achieve when acquiring a 3D volume or slab. The longer blood remains in the imaging volume, the lower its signal intensity due to repeated excitation and saturation effects. Increasing the TR or reducing the flip angle reduces such saturation effects. At the point of entry, the blood is fully magnetized. Higher flip angles generate much larger signal and contrast than lower flip angles. But the rate at which the signal from flowing blood approaches a suppressed steady state also is much greater. Therefore, there is much less depth penetration at higher flip angles, but flow will have greater signal at the point of entry. Conversely, with lower flip angles, the vessel signal and contrast at the slab entry are much less, but likewise approach a suppressed steady state much more slowly, thereby allowing for better depth penetration. These are major trade-offs in the selection of imaging parameters for 3D TOF MRA. Fig. **43–1A,B** presents MIP images from two circle of Willis 3D TOF MRA exams, illustrating a flip angle of 75° in Fig. **43–1A** and 25° in Fig. **43–1B**. Saturation effects (arrows, Fig. **43–1A**) are noted at the distal edges of the slabs (in this three-part multislab exam) when a too high tip angle is employed. To further complicate matters, techniques also exist in which the flip angle is varied across the imaging volume to more fully utilize the available magnetization and lessen saturation effects.

One major technique that is used to reduce the signal from background tissue and thereby increase the contrast between the background and flowing blood is magnetization transfer (MT). A short explanation of MT follows (see also case 56). There are two basic pools of hydrogen (protons) in the body. The "free" pool consists of the water molecules as a whole. The "bound" pool is not composed of water molecules

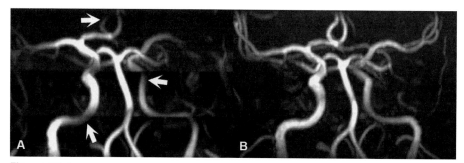

Figure 43–1

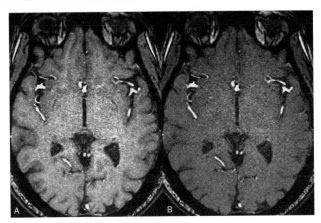

Figure 43–2

but rather of hydrogen nuclei bound to macromolecules. The tightly bound, or restricted, protons tumble slowly and have an extremely short T2 (and are thus not visualized by conventional MR, because the signal decays too rapidly). Additionally, they resonate over a broad frequency range. MT techniques use a special pulse to ex-

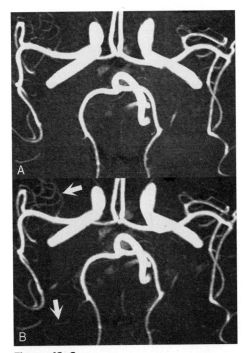

Figure 43–3

cite some of the restricted protons, which then transfer their magnetization to free water protons. The net result is a reduction in signal intensity (SI) from the free water. The amount of signal reduction depends on the makeup of the tissue with respect to the "bound" and "free" pool, as well as the method used to apply the MT pulse. The more macromolecules and long-chain protein molecules there are, the greater the effect of MT in that voxel. For gray and white matter, applying an MT pulse can reduce the signal intensity by up to 40%. Reducing the MR signal from background tissue can greatly improve vessel contrast on an MRA study. Fig. **43–2A** was acquired without MT and Fig. **43–2B** with MT. Note the reduction in signal intensity from brain with MT. Fig. **43–3** illustrates the corresponding MIPs. Note the improved visualization of small vessels in the MT image (white arrows, Fig. **43–3B**).

44   2D Phase Contrast MRA

Phase contrast (PC) MRA techniques rely on velocity-induced phase shifts to distinguish between flowing and stationary protons. Flow-encoding gradients are used to sensitize the image to flow. Phase contrast sequences can be acquired in either a 2D or 3D fashion; the discussion that follows focuses on 2D. Phase contrast images can be displayed as phase images (Fig. **44–1A,B**), where flow sensitivity is a function of direction, or as magnitude images (Fig. **44–1C,D**), where all vessels with flowing blood are bright, regardless of flow direction.

As blood flows along the direction of a gradient magnetic field from a lower to higher field, it increases in frequency (or gains phase) relative to stationary tissue. If

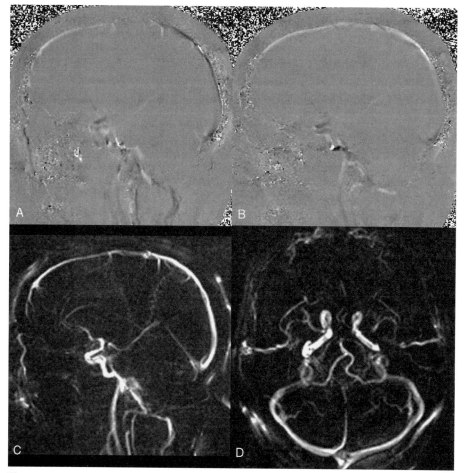

Figure 44–1

flowing in the opposite direction, it decreases in frequency (or loses phase). The amount of phase shift depends on the velocity of flow as well as the amplitude and duration of the flow-encoding gradients. Because blood flow can be in any direction, depending on the orientation of the vessel, flow-encoding gradients are applied in either one or all three orthogonal planes (x, y, and/or z). The choice of one or all directions is user selectable. Stationary tissue does not have any phase shift, and thus is not depicted on phase contrast images. Two types of images are generated with phase contrast sequences: phase images, in which the pixel intensity (i.e., bright or dark) relates to the direction of flow (Fig. **44–1A,B**) and magnitude images, in which the pixel intensity relates to flow velocity (Fig. **44–1C,D**).

One of the major advantages of PC techniques is the ability to choose the velocity to which the acquisition will be sensitive (i.e., slow or fast flow). The parameter selected by the operator is the velocity encoding (VENC). The image displayed in Fig. **44–1C** is a single 40-mm-thick slice (slab) acquired using a VENC of 20 cm/sec. Using that VENC, blood protons flowing 20 cm/sec accumulate the maximum phase shift ($-180°$ to $+180°$) and therefore are shown with the highest pixel intensity. Protons flowing slower as well as faster than the VENC exhibit less pixel intensity. The magnitude images from the different flow-encoding directions can be combined to form a single image, the "magnitude sum." The images in Fig. **44–1C,D** are, in fact, magnitude sum images.

In certain situations, one may wish to ascertain the direction of flow. In phase images, blood protons flowing along the direction of the flow-encoding gradient are reconstructed as white, and those flowing counter to the encoding gradient are reconstructed as black. In Fig. **44–1A**, the flow-encoding gradient is inferior to superior. As such, blood flowing within the anterior portion of superior sagittal sinus is bright. Blood flowing in the posterior portion is black because it is flowing counter to the direction of encoding. In Fig. **44–1B**, the flow-encoding gradient is anterior to posterior. It is important to remember that if blood is flowing faster than the selected VENC, then it will experience greater than 180° of phase shift and will appear to the reconstruction algorithm to be flowing in the opposite direction (phase aliasing). PC sequences are a good choice for imaging the venous structures of the head and neck and for acquiring quick "scout" images of the vessels in the neck. Alternatively, for depiction of venous structures, 2D time-of-flight MRA can be employed (see case 41).

45 Contrast-Enhanced MRA: Basics (Renal, Abdomen)

The contrast-enhanced MRA maximum intensity projection (MIP) image displayed in Fig. **45–1A** demonstrates moderate to severe stenosis at the origin of the left renal artery (arrow). Fig. **45–1B** demonstrates extensive atherosclerotic disease involving the aorta, with severe stenosis at the origin of the left renal artery. The study presented in Fig. **45–1C–F** depicts a high-grade stenosis (arrow) involving the right renal artery, with Fig. **45–1D** and Fig. **45–1E** being coronal and axial source images and Fig. **45–1F** a targeted MIP, confirmed on catheter angiography (Fig. **45–1G**).

Contrast-enhanced MRA (CE-MRA) is fast becoming routine in evaluation of the abdominal aorta and renal arteries. The standard imaging sequence is a fast 3D spoiled gradient echo sequence. Thin sections (on the order of 2 mm or less) are acquired in the coronal plane within a breath hold (typically 30 seconds or less), using a very short TR and TE. Acquiring a 3D volume in such a fashion results in a high degree of saturation (low MR signal) of the background tissues as well as the blood within the vessels. Bolus injection of a gadolinium chelate leads to a substantial reduction in the T1 relaxation time of blood, producing images with very high signal intensity vascular structures, due to the gadolinium chelate "enhanced" blood within. Typically 30 to 40 mL of contrast media is injected at a rate of 1.5 to 3 mL/second. The bolus of contrast agent is immediately followed by a bolus of normal saline, typically 20 to 30 mL injected at the same rate. The purpose of the saline is to maintain the contrast in a tight bolus as it travels through the vascular system.

In every MR acquisition, and of particular relevance for CE-MRA, the raw data (as sampled) occupies k space, the coordinates of which are frequency and phase as opposed to x and y. High spatial frequency data, found in the periphery of k space, contains information regarding predominantly image detail. Low spatial frequency data, found in the center of k space, contains information regarding predominantly image (tissue) contrast. The position of data in k space is determined by the amplitude of the phase encoding gradient applied prior to sampling of the echo (MR signal). Echoes acquired during the application of high-amplitude gradients contain principally information regarding spatial resolution. Echoes acquired during the application of low-amplitude gradients contain principally information regarding tissue contrast (as well as containing most of the observed signal). CE-MRA acquisitions are timed such that the acquisition of the central lines of k space coincides with the maximum concentration of contrast media (gadolinium chelate) in the area of interest.

It is therefore very important to know both the circulation time to the area of interest and the order in which the k-space data is collected. Most systems allow the operator to select the order of k-space filling. Typical terminology used refers to the filling of the central portion first as "centric" and the filling of the outer lines first as "linear."

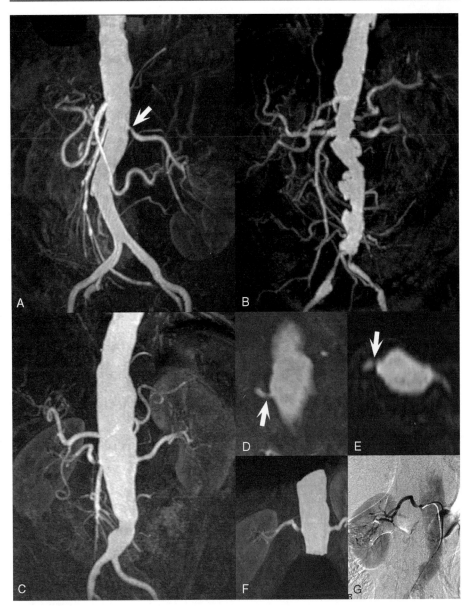

Figure 45–1

46 Contrast-Enhanced MRA: Carotid Arteries

A maximum intensity projection (MIP) of the entire data set (Fig. **46–1A**) from a contrast-enhanced MRA of the carotids reveals the aortic arch, origin of the great vessels, carotid arteries, and vertebrobasilar system. There is nonvisualization of the right internal carotid artery, with occlusion of this vessel at its origin. The MIP image is created following completion of the scan from source images, which are usually acquired in the coronal plane. In many instances a data set is acquired both immediately prior to and during contrast injection, with the first set of images serving as a mask (and the MIP image created from the subtraction of the two data sets). Sample source images (from the 80 images that constituted the coronal slab) are also illustrated (mask and with contrast, Fig. **46–1B,C**). Targeted MIP reconstructions, in which only the carotid arteries are included, confirm occlusion (*) of the right internal carotid artery at its origin (Fig. **46–1D**) and display clearly the focal severe stenosis of the left internal carotid artery at its origin (arrow, Fig. **46–1E**).

Contrast-enhanced MRA (CE-MRA) of the carotid arteries offers several advantages over conventional 2D or 3D time-of-flight (TOF) techniques. In TOF acquisitions, a thin slice (2D) or a slab (3D) is excited using a relatively short TR. This results in saturation of (reduced signal from) background tissue. "Fresh" unsaturated blood flowing into the slice or slab has not been exposed to an RF pulse and thus has high signal intensity. TOF techniques produce images based on this flow-related enhancement. Problems arise when there is turbulent flow, reversal of flow, higher orders of motion (acceleration), or very slow flow. Any of these conditions can result in loss of signal within a vessel. These complex flow patterns occur in both normal as well as diseased vessels, which historically resulted in overestimation of the degree of stenoses. With CE-MRA techniques, the image contrast is based on T1 differences between background tissue and the gadolinium chelate "enhanced" blood. This, together with the very short echo time (TE) typically used, greatly reduces the artifactual signal loss due to complex flow patterns and allows for excellent visualization of the arterial system. The use of a coronal 3D slab permits improved craniocaudal coverage without impacting scan time (as demonstrated in Fig. **46–1A**). It should be noted, however, that a larger field of view suffers from poorer spatial resolution, in general, when compared with a smaller field of view.

Another advantage of CE-MRA is reduced scan times. In this patient case, the scan time was 19 seconds compared with several minutes for TOF techniques. In addition, 2D TOF sequences acquire slices in a sequential fashion, with swallowing motion producing severe misregistration artifacts. In a rapid 3D acquisition (as used for CE-MRA), swallowing artifacts (if even present) are distributed over the entire data set and are essentially not an issue.

The order of k-space sampling (typically chosen to be centric) and the timing of image acquisition are crucial for CE-MRA of the carotid arteries. The transit time of the contrast bolus from the common carotid arteries to the jugular veins can be as fast as 6 to 7 seconds, with little margin for error in timing the acquisition to avoid venous contamination.

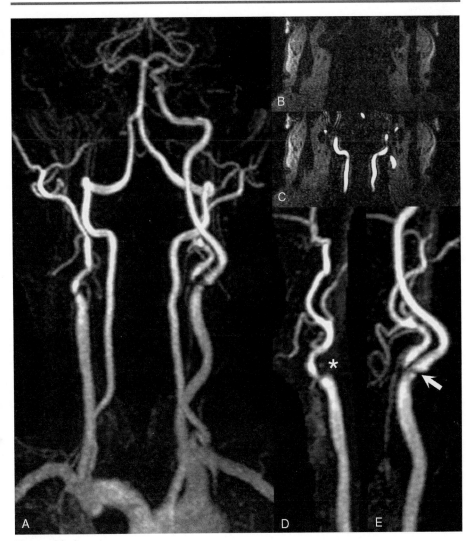

Figure 46–1

47 Contrast-Enhanced MRA: Peripheral Circulation

Fig. **47–1A** illustrates 3D contrast-enhanced MR angiography (CE-MRA) of the lower extremities, in a patient with no significant stenoses or occlusions. The adjacent 3D CE-MRA examination of the femoropopliteal distribution (Fig. **47–1B**) reveals, in a different patient, bilateral superficial femoral artery occlusion with development of profunda femoral artery collaterals. Fig. **47–1C,D** are multiphase CE-MRA images of the tibioperoneal distribution obtained during early arterial enhancement and (with a slight time delay) after substantial venous filling. In the latter image, the large vascular malformation in the left gastrocnemius is more completely visualized, due to opacification of the venous component.

Peripheral MRA may be performed in three ways: time-of-flight (TOF) (see cases 41 and 42), phase contrast (see case 44), and contrast enhanced (CE). The latter technique has become popular due to the short scan time and, more importantly, because its sensitivity and specificity approach that of traditional x-ray angiography for peripheral vascular disease. Peripheral 3D CE-MRA utilizes short TR/short TE 3D gradient echo sequences, obtained in three to four stations in the coronal plane. Automated table positioning is incorporated with image acquisition through all stations. Timing is set so that the scan is acquired during passage of the gadolinium chelate bolus, or equivalently during maximal contrast concentration within the vessel of interest. Detection of T1 shortening and therefore the start of image acquisition occur via one of four methods: (1) A test bolus may be used to approximate the timing of bolus arrival during the actual examination. (2) In MR fluoroscopy, rapid 2D scans allow the technologist to monitor for arrival of the contrast bolus and thereby manually initiate the 3D CE-MRA scan (used for Fig. **47–1A,B**). (3) In multiphase CE-MRA (Fig. **47–1C,D**), rapid time sequential 3D scans are acquired, permitting dynamic imaging of the passage of contrast through the arterial and venous circulation. (4) Automated bolus detection algorithms involve computer detection of bolus arrival and initiation of image acquisition.

The center of k space (see case 10), which is the major determinant of image contrast, must be obtained when arterial enhancement is at its peak (not on the up-slope as this increases ring artifact) and venous enhancement is at a minimum. At station 1 (aortoiliac), the center of k space is obtained near either the midpoint or end of the scan to ensure that data acquisition occurs during arterial enhancement (with the scan initiated when contrast is first visualized in the proximal aorta). This order of acquisition is "reversed" in station 2 (femoropopliteal) and station 3 (tibioperoneal) or station 3 alone. The center of k space in this station(s) is obtained during the beginning of the scan via centric phase reordering, assuring that this portion of the scan is acquired during peak arterial enhancement.

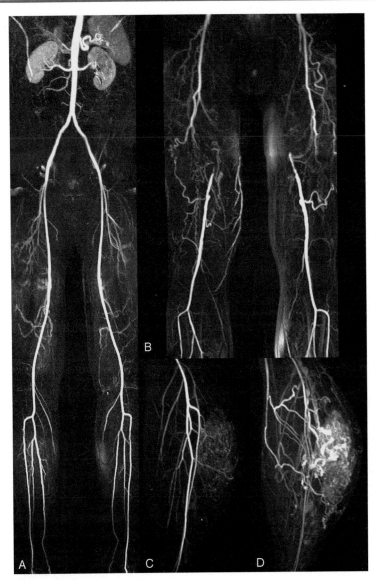

Figure 47–1

48 Abdomen: Motion Correction (Part 1)

There are currently four major methods available to compensate for respiratory organ displacement:

1. Simply ask patients to hold their breath.
2. Trigger the scan using the signals from a respiratory belt.
3. Trace the respiratory cycle using a "navigator" echo, selecting or rejecting acquired data.
4. Trace the respiratory cycle using a navigator echo, adjusting the slice position following the respiratory organ displacement.

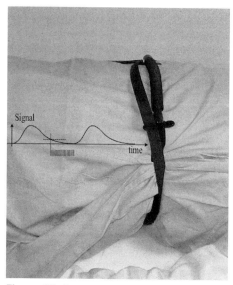

Figure 48–1

As indicated in Fig. **48–1,** the signal from the respiratory belt can be used to start the acquisition of the imaging sequence close to either inspiration or expiration. A more current and elegant solution is to trace the motion of the liver–lung interface with a so-called navigator echo (Fig. **48–2**).

Some vendors call this approach PACE (prospective acquisition correction). For the navigator echo, a "rod of tissue" is excited, placed through the dome of the liver with a one-dimensional craniocaudal extension (Fig. **48–2A**). The one-dimensional information is read out in parallel to the imaging sequence with the motion of the liver–lung interface serving as an indicator for breathing (Fig. **48–2B**). The user can define whether data acquisition should be activated close to the inspiratory or expiratory portion of the respiratory cycle. Usually a tolerance in millimeters of liver excursion is taken as an indication of whether the data acquisition is to be switched on or off.

Fig. **48–3A,B** presents fast spin echo T2-weighted images in a patient with multiple hemangiomas acquired using PACE. Fig. **48–3C,D** presents fast spin echo magnitude inversion recovery images of the same region, also using PACE. For steady-state sequences, the RF and gradient application is continuously applied, whereas it is the data collection that is "gated." Alternatively, to increase the number of valid data points acquired for a given time, the observed shift of the diaphragm can simply be used to correct the position of excitation, following spatially the shift in craniocaudal position of intraabdominal organs with respiration.

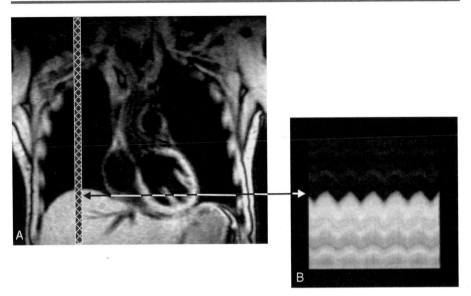

Figure 48–2

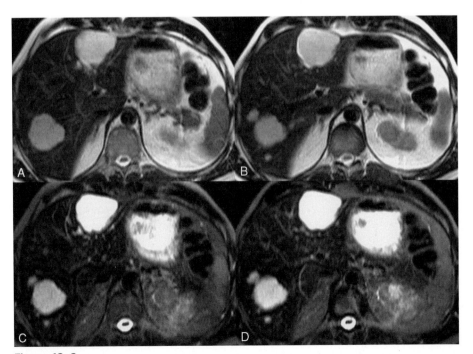

Figure 48–3

49 Abdomen: Motion Correction (Part 2)

Magnetic resonance provides an excellent tool for imaging of the internal structures of the thorax and abdomen. However, physiologic motion (for example, respiration and cardiac pulsation) can lead to artifacts, reducing the diagnostic quality of the final image. Most MR scanners offer hardware, software, and sequence-based options designed to minimize or eliminate the effects of physiologic motion during scan acquisition.

Motion artifacts in MR images are caused by translations or shifts in the position of the imaged structure during the acquisition of data. Routine spin echo and gradient echo sequences encode and acquire data to fill k space in a line-by-line fashion, with the collection of each line separated by a certain amount of time (TR). In fast spin echo imaging, several, but not all, lines are collected with each TR. Because all the data for an entire slice are not acquired simultaneously, changes in the location of anatomic structures between TR periods can lead to misalignment in spatial encoding. Fourier transform of the lines of k space data results in blurring or ghosting (see case 98) in the final image (Fig. **49–1**), the well-recognized consequences of motion during scan acquisition.

The simplest and most effective method of respiratory motion reduction is to have patients hold their breath. Rapidly acquired T1- and T2-weighted gradient echo sequences are used to collect data during suspended respiration, thereby minimizing motion artifacts. However, this approach requires the scan time to be 25 seconds or less for the average patient, leading to limitations in spatial resolution and number of slices. The use of this approach is also restricted by the patients' health and mental status, as well as their age.

Single slice techniques such as HASTE, trueFISP, and echo planar imaging acquire the data for one entire slice before beginning the next slice. In most cases, the acquisition is rapid enough to freeze respiratory motion, greatly minimizing artifacts within each slice. This method, however, does not account for changes in anatomic position between slices. The addition of techniques such as gating or breath holding is necessary to assure consistent and complete anatomic coverage.

Respiratory gating (see case 48) incorporates the use of a bellows device placed around the patient's chest to track respiratory motion. Data are acquired during a specific portion of the respiratory cycle defined in the sequence parameters during setup. This method can greatly reduce respiratory artifacts; however, scan times are lengthened by up to a factor of three.

The use of navigator echoes is an important alternative for reduction of respiratory related image artifacts, which does not require either additional hardware or patient cooperation. The simplest, one-dimensional navigator involves additional RF pulses in the sequence to track superior to inferior translational motion of abdominal and thoracic structures based on the diaphragmatic position. Information from the navigator echo can be used to trigger data acquisition during a specified portion of the respiratory cycle or to adjust the anatomic (craniocaudal) position of a slice group to follow the change occurring during respiration. Higher order navigator echoes also

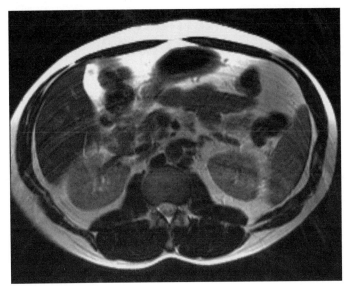

Figure 49–1

exist to adjust for two-dimensional translation in cardiac imaging and three-dimensional translation in the brain during functional MRI studies.

Incorporating navigators to reduce the time required for breath holding involves breaking up large, multislice measurements into smaller groups of slices, reducing the breath hold duration of each group by a corresponding amount. Differences in the diaphragmatic position between measurements due to varying levels of inspiratory volume are corrected by gradient system adjustments, reducing the chance for overlapping of slices or large gaps in slice coverage.

50 Volume Interpolated Breath-Hold Examination (VIBE)

The outer lines of k space contain information about the details within the image, the high spatial frequencies. In these outer k-space lines, the transverse magnetization of adjacent voxels points in opposite directions. For a homogeneous phantom, having the transverse magnetization point in opposite directions for adjacent voxels means that the net magnetization is zero and no signal is induced. For a heterogeneous object, there is some signal, although it is very small. Omitting the data collection of those small signals causes truncation artifacts (see case 103). Filling these data lines with zero values (as in Fig. **50–1B**), will greatly improve the image appearance. Fig. **50–1A** illustrates the situation in which all k-space lines are acquired in a 3D scan. In Fig. **50–1B**, only the more central lines along the slice gradient axis are acquired. It would be incorrect to believe that images interpolated in this way are identical to what would have been obtained if the object had been scanned with a full k-space acquisition. On the other hand, the zero-filling approach, as implemented with the volume interpolated breath-hold examination (VIBE) technique, does improve the partial volume effect. In other words, zero filling does not improve spatial or volume resolution, but it does reduce the artifacts caused by the shape and size of pixels in the image.

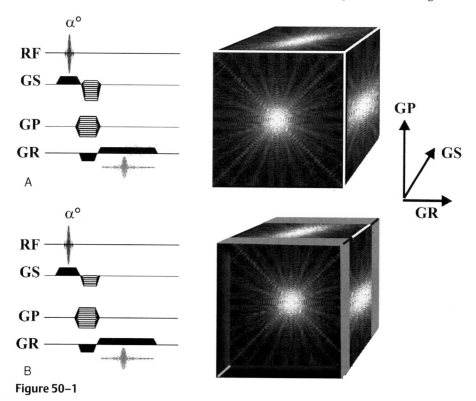

Figure 50–1

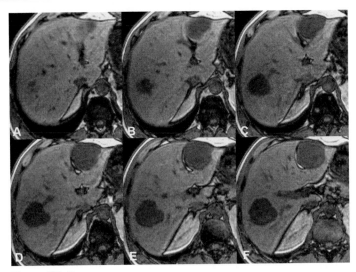

Figure 50–2

Fig. **50–2** presents images from a 3D T1-weighted gradient echo acquisition in a patient with multiple liver hemangiomas. The slice thickness was 5 mm. Fig. **50–3** is using the same technique, but with Fourier interpolation, providing 3-mm cuts through the same pathology in the same measurement time with the same anatomic coverage. Note the larger number of images that cover the same anatomic region within the liver, comparing Fig. **50–3** to Fig. **50–2** (due to the 3-mm as opposed to 5-mm slice thickness). In clinical practice, VIBE is used for acquisition of dynamic postcontrast scans of the upper abdomen. It is typically implemented with fat suppression, using a 3D fast low-angle shot (FLASH) pulse sequence.

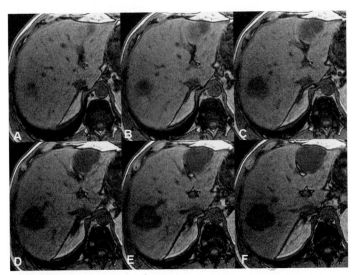

Figure 50–3

51 Magnetic Resonance Cholangiopancreatography (MRCP)

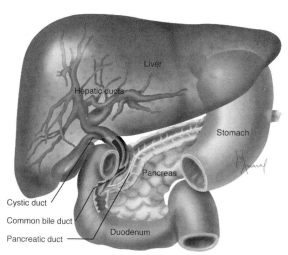

Magnetic resonance cholangiopancreatography (MRCP) is a noninvasive alternative for the visualization of the common bile, cystic, pancreatic, and hepatic ducts (Fig. 51-1) without instrumentation, ionizing radiation, or the administration of a contrast agent. The results are comparable to those obtained with endoscopic retrograde cholangiopancreatography (ERCP), without the complications that can occur following this invasive procedure.

Figure 51–1

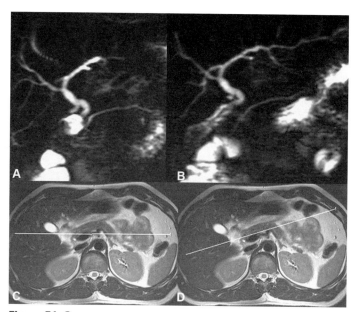

Figure 51–2

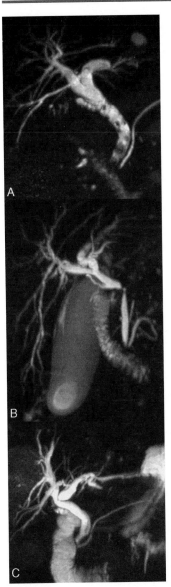

Figure 51–3

Specific MRCP techniques vary, but commonly consist of several rapid scans acquired during a routine abdominal MR exam. After anatomic localization, a thick slab, single-shot fast spin echo sequence (e.g., HASTE) with an echo time (TE) on the order of 1000 ms is acquired.

The high TE exploits the inherently long T2-relaxation time of some fluids, including bile. The transverse magnetization of surrounding tissues with comparatively short relaxation times fully decays before echo formation, leaving only the signal contribution from fluid to complete the image (Fig. **51–2A,B**). The sequence is run at multiple angles (Fig. **51–2C,D**) to provide the best view of the ducts (Fig. **51–2A,B**) and to remove residual bowel signal that can obscure ductal anatomy. A thin slice, single-shot sequence is then acquired, which provides high-resolution images for ductal analysis and 3D reconstruction. Recently, to obtain higher spatial resolution with greater anatomic coverage, 3D volume acquisitions have been used (Fig. **51–3**) (images courtesy of Richard Gregory, Gold Coast Hospital, Queensland, Australia). These sequences take longer to acquire and incorporate navigator echoes, with data acquisition triggered according to the position of the diaphragm to reduce anatomic misregistration caused by respiration.

Fig. **51–3** illustrates 3D MRCP exams from three patients, all with biliary obstruction and enlargement. The level of obstruction and cause differs by patient, with multiple stones noted within the common bile duct in Fig. **51–3A**, as compared with obstruction along the midportion in Fig. **51–3B** and terminus in Fig. **51–3C** of the common bile duct.

Patient preparation is not necessary for MRCP on a routine basis; however, fluid in the stomach and small bowel may obscure important anatomic structures. Negative bowel agents such as ferric ammonium citrate or blueberry juice, the latter being rich in manganese, have proven successful in the suppression of the signal produced by gastric and duodenal fluids. High spatial resolution and the use of single shot sequences as well as navigator techniques make MRCP an effective replacement to ERCP for visualization of the pancreatic and biliary ductal anatomy.

52 Fat Suppression: Spectral Saturation

The suppression of signal produced by adipose tissue in MRI can be helpful in the delineation and differentiation of certain tissues and pathologies. An often-preferred method for accomplishing this task is spectral fat saturation. Fig. **52–1** presents axial T1-weighted images of the upper abdomen without (Fig. **52–1A**) and with (Fig. **52–1B**) spectral fat saturation, respectively. Note that the pancreas (arrow) is well delineated (and slightly hyperintense) on the image with fat saturation, leading to widespread use of this technique for pancreatic imaging.

In vivo, water and fat protons resonate at slightly different frequencies in a magnetic field. This frequency separation increases with field strength. The difference at 1.5 T is ~220 Hz, as shown in Fig. **52–1C**. A specially designed RF pulse is applied prior

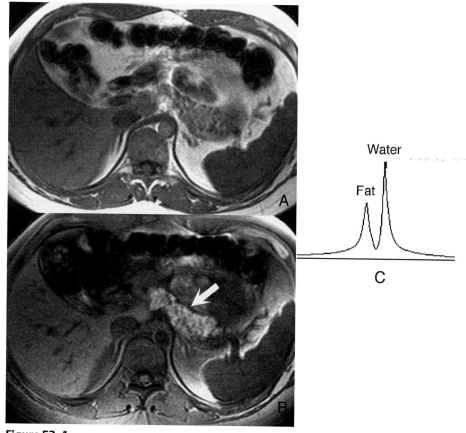

Figure 52–1

to the spin preparation excitation at the specific resonance frequency of fat, which saturates the spins at this frequency. The fat tissue within the field of view remains saturated during the spin excitation and therefore does not contribute to the resulting echo and image formation.

The presence of ferromagnetic objects or large variations in tissue shape (e.g., neck and chest) within the volume of interest can substantially affect magnetic susceptibility (see case 93), leading to a change in the specific resonant frequency of fat in localized areas. Advanced MR systems are equipped with special hardware, called electronic shims, that produce small changes in the spatial magnetic field to optimize the homogeneity within the field of view. The result is greater uniformity of the magnetic field with less chance for incomplete or inconsistent fat saturation. Regardless, users should make an extra effort to assure that all metal objects, including buttons and jewelry, are removed prior to the exam to improve the final spectral fat saturation.

Spectral fat saturation is often also employed in the lumbar spine to facilitate the detection of lesions within the marrow on T2-weighted scans. Fig. **52–2** presents sagittal T2-weighted images of the lumbar spine without (Fig. **52–2A**) and with (Fig. **52–2B**) spectral fat saturation, respectively. Note the improved visualization of disk hydration (and the loss of hydration at L5-S1, arrow) in the image with fat saturation.

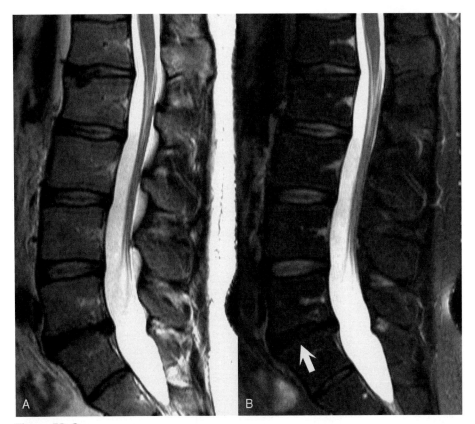

Figure 52–2

53 Water Excitation, Fat Excitation

As outlined previously, the different electronic environment of water-bound and fat-bound hydrogen atoms means that their respective magnetic moments (of the hydrogen nuclei) precess at different resonance frequencies. The magnetic moments of hydrogen nuclei in adipose tissue have a resonance frequency that is ~3.5 ppm lower than that within water-containing tissue. A frequency selective saturation pulse can thus be used to suppress the signal from adipose tissue. The quality of that saturation is a function of the overall homogeneity within the imaging volume. In addition, the fat saturating RF pulse is usually very close to the water resonance, resulting in an overall loss in signal-to-noise ratio (SNR). As an alternative, it is theoretically possible to simply excite either water or fat in the absence of a magnetic field gradient, employing only the small, corresponding frequency range. In practice such an approach tends to be prone to artifacts because it requires excellent field homogeneity within the volume of interest. Better results for water or fat excitation have been achieved with so-called binomial pulses (1-1, 1-2-1, or 1-3-3-1). Fig. **53–1** illustrates the use of

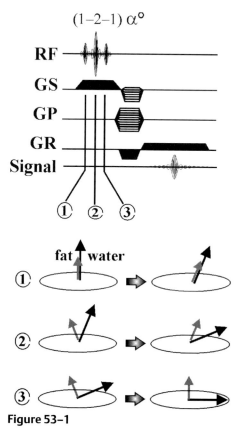

a slice-selective 1-2-1 binomial pulse for water excitation. To achieve a 90° excitation for water, there is an initial 22.5° excitation pulse. A waiting period allows the slower rotating transverse magnetization within adipose tissue to develop a phase difference, for example, 180° with respect to the phase position of the transverse magnetization within water. The 45° excitation angle then tips the magnetization within water to 67.5° with respect to the longitudinal direction, whereas the magnetization within adipose tissue is flipped to 22.5° in the same direction. After the waiting period, a further 22.5° excitation pulse completes the 90° excitation for water, with the magnetization of fat restored to the longitudinal position and thus not contributing to the MR signal. The net result is a "water excitation" RF pulse. Using the same approach, but with a phase shift (of the RF pulse), a "fat excitation" pulse can be created if desired. By exciting selectively either fat or water, only the excited tissue produces an MR signal in the final image. Nonselective RF pulses can be used if the organ is small enough or the transmit coil excites only

Figure 53–1

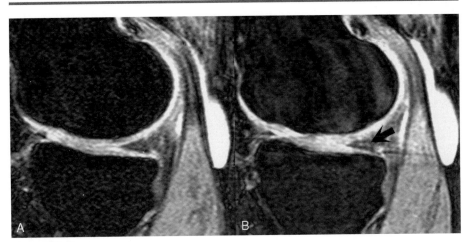

Figure 53–2

a small region, allowing phase encoding in two orthogonal directions within an acceptable measurement time (3D acquisition). Binomial pulses that are slice or slab selective are referred to as spectral spatial pulses.

Sagittal images of the knee are presented in Fig. **53–2** from a patient with a small popliteal (Baker's) cyst. Fig. **53–2A** was acquired using a refocused GRE [fast imaging with steady precession (FISP)] sequence with a spectral fat saturation pulse. Fig. **53–2B** was acquired with the same pulse sequence, but using a composite pulse for water excitation rather than spectral fat saturation. The image acquired with water excitation, despite the inadvertent superimposed motion artifact, has better SNR and provides improved visualization of the abnormal intrameniscal signal (arrow, Fig. **53–2B**), which is due to degenerative meniscal disease.

54 Fat Suppression: Short Tau Inversion Recovery (STIR)

In inversion recovery imaging, suppression of the signal from adipose tissue can be achieved by exploiting the short T1-relaxation time of fat. The sequence starts with a 180° pulse, which tips the longitudinal magnetization antiparallel to the main magnetic field direction. Immediately after this inversion, the longitudinal magnetization begins to relax back to the equilibrium orientation, parallel to the main magnetic field. The time necessary for this process depends on the tissue-specific T1 relaxation time. The time between the center of the inversion pulse and the center of the excitation pulse of the imaging sequence is called the inversion time (TI). The longitudinal magnetization within fat tissue has a very short relaxation time, on the order of 130 to 170 ms. The longitudinal magnetization of fat, on crossing from a negative to a positive value, passes through zero. If the excitation pulse of the imaging sequence is applied at that point in time, little or no transverse magnetization is generated and only a small or no MR signal is detected from fat (Fig. **54–1**).

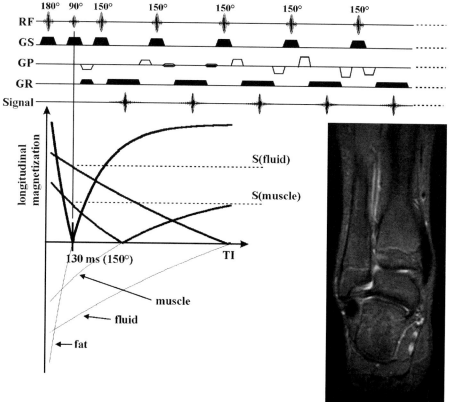

Figure 54–1

Because the inversion time of 130 to 170 ms was called a "short tau" in the early days of MRI, the term *short tau inversion recovery* (STIR) remained. STIR imaging is usually performed in conjunction with a fast spin echo sequence, to take advantage of the shorter measurement time possible with fast spin echo imaging. When combined with longer repetition times and higher matrix sizes, better contrast and spatial resolution is obtained in comparison with a conventional spin echo sequence. STIR is an inversion recovery technique that generally produces magnitude images that provide no information about the sign of the longitudinal magnetization. Consequently, tissues with short relaxation times may appear bright, in common with tissues having longer relaxation times. As indicated in Fig. **54–1,** the signal from fluid is proportional to the available longitudinal magnetization and is significantly higher than the signal from muscle. Adipose tissue has no signal contribution, provided that the inversion time and amplitude of the inversion pulse have been adjusted appropriately. STIR images have an intrinsically low SNR, because most of the longitudinal magnetization is still oriented antiparallel to the main magnetic field and is far from being fully relaxed.

STIR in conjunction with T1-shortening contrast agents (e.g., the gadolinium chelates) has to be used with caution. Contrast uptake in a lesion is unlikely to lead to signal enhancement but rather to a lower signal in STIR images, because the longitudinal magnetization does not recover fast enough from its large antiparallel alignment to an equivalent parallel alignment to the main magnetic field direction.

As illustrated in Fig. **54–1,** STIR imaging has the potential to reveal any fluid accumulation within bone marrow, around joints, and along tendon sheaths (including soft tissue and marrow edema). Blood vessels appear hyperintense. Because fat suppression with STIR does not depend on local field homogeneity, it serves as an alternative to spectral fat saturation in intrinsically inhomogeneous body regions, for example, the orbits.

55 Fat Suppression: Phase Cycling

The two hydrogen-based longitudinal magnetizations used in MRI have their origins in adipose (fat) and water-containing tissue. Due to the different electronic environment in adipose tissue, the resonance frequency of that magnetization is ~3.5 ppm lower than that of water (~ −220 Hz on a 1.5-T system, as previously noted). With time, after the initial excitation (Fig. **55–1**), the transverse magnetization within adipose tissue falls behind the transverse magnetization within water. The time of the gradient echo—specifically, when the MR signal is observed—can be chosen so that the transverse magnetizations from fat and water are either opposed-phase or in-phase.

The duration of the acquisition window in a pulse sequence is inversely proportional to the bandwidth of the sequence. If the bandwidth is large enough (and thus the acquisition window very short), it is possible to acquire opposed-phase and in-phase images simultaneously with a double echo gradient echo sequence (Fig. **55–1**). This approach is typically employed with TE, TR, and tip angle chosen to provide T1-weighting. Thus, voxels containing fat are high signal intensity and those containing water are low signal intensity. However, in voxels in which there is both fat and water, on opposed-phase images, there is a cancellation (loss) of signal due to the transverse magnetization from fat and water being of opposite phase. This leads to signal loss at the interface between fat- and water-containing structures, for example at the margin of the liver (or spleen) and adjacent intraabdominal fat.

Illustrated in Fig. **55–2** is a nonhyperfunctioning adrenal adenoma, on Fig. **55–2A** in-phase and on Fig. **55–2B** opposed-phase images (reprinted with permission from Runge VM, ed. *Clinical Magnetic Resonance Imaging.* Philadelphia: WB Saunders; 2002). A round, sharply demarcated, homogeneous lesion of the left adrenal gland is

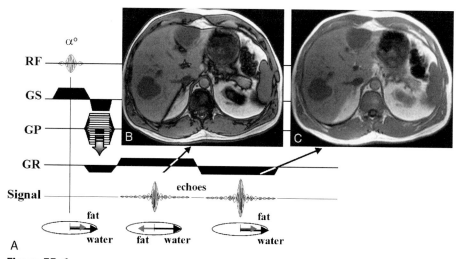

A

Figure 55–1

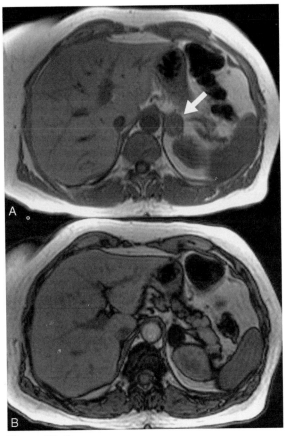

noted (arrow). On the in-phase image, the lesion is nearly isointense with normal liver parenchyma. On the opposed-phase image, the lesion is markedly hypointense. This illustrates one of the major clinical applications of opposed-phase imaging. Eighty percent of adrenal adenomas contain sufficient lipid to show a marked signal intensity reduction on opposed-phase imaging, which is not seen for the other major lesions considered in the differential diagnosis: metastasis, pheochromocytoma, and adrenal carcinoma.

Figure 55–2

56 Magnetization Transfer

iced tea

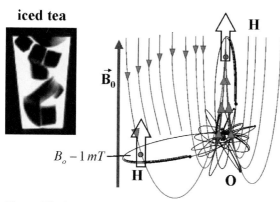

$\vec{B_0}$

$B_o - 1\,mT$

H

H

O

Figure 56–1

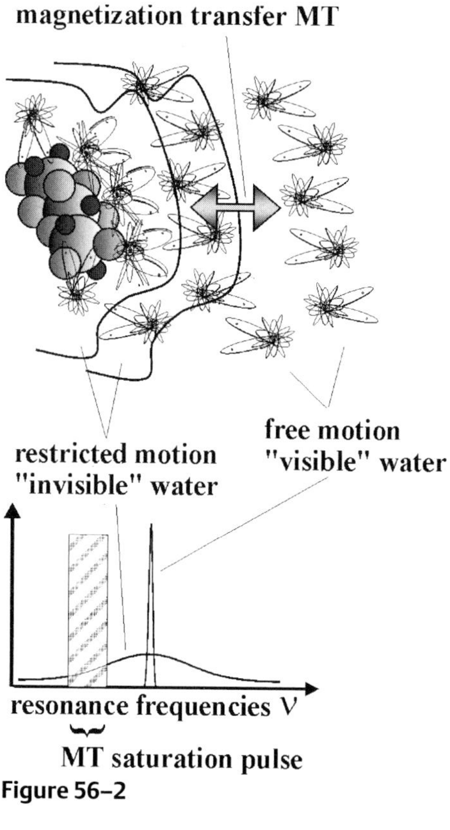

magnetization transfer MT

restricted motion
"invisible" water

free motion
"visible" water

resonance frequencies ν

MT saturation pulse

Figure 56–2

As illustrated in Fig. **56–1**, the magnetic moment of one hydrogen nucleus, if aligned parallel to the magnetic field, superimposes its own intrinsic field on its neighbor. Depending on the orientation of the water molecule (which contains two hydrogen nuclei) within the main magnetic field, the field strength at that location will be increased or decreased. Because the number of possible orientations is large, there is also a large range of different resonance frequencies. The latter causes the sum of all magnetizations, the transverse magnetization, to dephase rapidly. The T2 relaxation time can be as short as 10 µs. Water molecules that are frozen in their orientation are not visible (due to the very short T2). Ice cubes within the iced tea thus appear hypointense (Fig. **56–1**).

Due to the rapid tumbling motion of water molecules in the free ("visible") water pool, the magnetic field superimposed by adjacent hydrogen nuclei is averaged out. The resonance frequencies are found in a small range, resulting in a long T2 relaxation time. An "invisible" or restricted water pool also exists, due to hydrogen bound to complex macromolecules. MRI is unable to image the restricted pool due to its extremely short T2 values.

Placing a frequency selective saturation pulse below the resonance frequency of free water (Fig. **56–2**) results in a portion of the restricted water pool being saturated. Any transferred magnetization depends on the status of the magnetization within both pools. The restricted pool has short T1 relaxation times due to the effective rigid lattice condition and a very short T2 relaxation time. The short T1 relaxation time of the restricted pool indirectly influences the observed T1 relaxation time of the free and visible water pool. The magnetization transfer (MT) from the restricted to the unrestricted pool results not only in a decrease in magnetization, but also in a decrease in the observed relaxation times. Magnetization transfer thus provides an additional contrast mechanism influencing the signal intensity of tissue above and beyond the contrast provided by the spin density and T1 and T2 differences between tissues. Clinically, MT is used in MR angiography and for postcontrast T1-weighted imaging. In 3D time-of-flight (TOF) MR angiography, MT provides an improvement in vessel depiction, due to greater background tissue suppression. The use of MT in this instance also leads to (relative) higher signal intensity from fat (for example, in the orbits), which can degrade the study unless appropriately excluded by postprocessing. On postcontrast scans with MT, there is an improvement in the conspicuity of enhancing lesions due to the reduction in signal of surrounding brain. On the postcontrast images presented without (Fig. **56–3A**) and with (Fig. **56–3B**) MT, the change in tissue contrast, particularly the basal ganglia, and the improved lesion enhancement (a metastasis, arrow) with MT are noted.

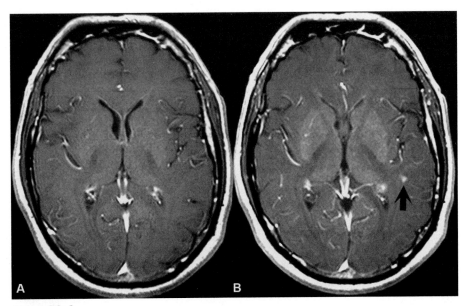

Figure 56–3

57 Calculating T1 and T2 Relaxation Times (Calculated Images)

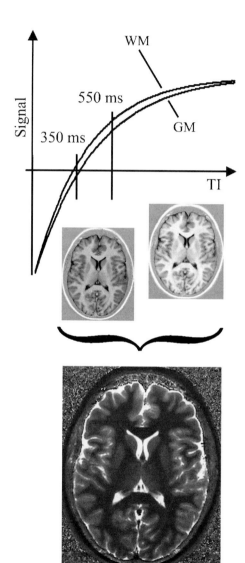

Figure 57–1

The classification of lesions based on their hypointense or hyperintense appearance is hampered by the influence of field strength and pulse sequence parameters. An alternative approach (but little used today clinically) is to calculate the tissue relaxation times, thus providing a quantitative means of tissue characterization. Inversion recovery (IR) imaging techniques are considered the most accurate approaches for the calculation of T1 relaxation times. A simple means of estimating T1 can be achieved by acquiring two images with different inversion times, in this example, 350 and 550 ms (Fig. **57–1**). The T1 value is then calculated based on these two points measured along the recovery path of the longitudinal magnetization. The resultant "calculated" image is displayed at the bottom of Fig. **57–1.** In this image, the value of each pixel corresponds to the T1 of the respective tissue, as opposed to arbitrary signal intensity as with the majority of MR images.

An alternative approach to the use of inversion recovery imaging is the acquisition of spin echo images with different T1-weighting (different repetition times, 550 and 950 ms in this instance). Based on the difference in signal intensity between the two acquisitions, the T1 value of the tissue can be estimated. It is important, however, that the change in signal intensity as a function of TR is well above the noise level of the image; otherwise, the calculated T1 image will be very noisy (as illustrated in Fig. **57–2**).

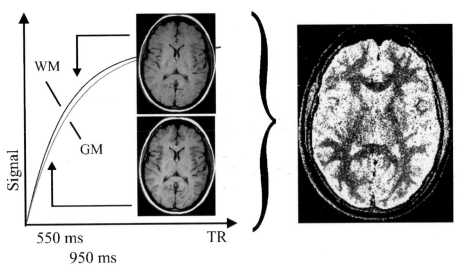

Figure 57-2

T2 relaxation times can be estimated from a single multi-echo measurement, where the echo time dependent signal decay follows the T2 relaxation time of the tissue. In Fig. **57-3,** three images with different echo times (TE) were acquired in a single multiecho scan. The change in signal intensity as a function of echo time is then used to generate a T2 pixel map, the final image shown in Fig. **57-3**.

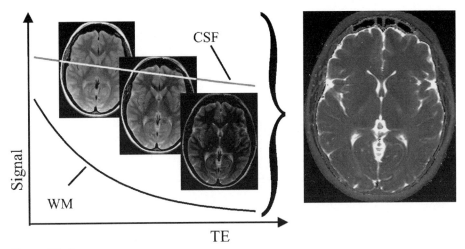

Figure 57-3

58 Perfusion Imaging

A watershed infarct between the middle and posterior cerebral artery territories is well visualized on fluid-attenuated inversion recovery (FLAIR) (Fig. **58–1A**) and diffusion-weighted (Fig. **58–1B**) images. The mean transit time (MTT) map (Fig. **58–1C**) reveals an overall pixel intensity increase and thus increased transit time

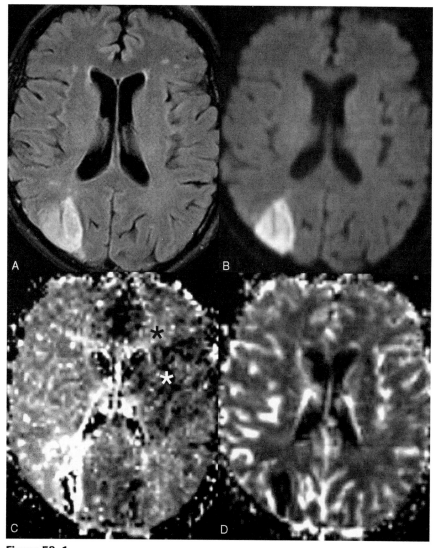

Figure 58–1

(slower arrival of the contrast agent bolus) within the area of the lesion, as well as the entire right cerebral hemisphere. The relative cerebral blood volume (rCBV) map (Fig. **58–1D**), however, shows little difference in the overall volume of blood between the right and left hemispheres, with the exception of the infarct itself.

Cerebral perfusion imaging is the visualization of changes or delays in microvascular blood flow in the brain. This imaging technique can be used to facilitate the evaluation of strokes, tumors, and the differentiation of radiation necrosis versus recurrent tumor. Perfusion imaging is made possible through the acquisition of multiple, time sequential, single-shot echo planar imaging (EPI) slices (see case 39) measured with a temporal resolution of 1 second or less during the rapid administration of a gadolinium chelate.

Today's high-end MR scanners with advanced gradient technology are able to accommodate coverage of the entire brain with slices acquired in a dynamic fashion immediately prior to, during, and following passage of the contrast bolus through the brain. The transit of a gadolinium chelate (as a concentrated, compact bolus) through the brain causes a decrease in tissue signal intensity on echo planar images due to the $T2^*$ or magnetic susceptibility effect of the agent. Using this acquired data, calculations are made to demonstrate the rate of change in the MR signal as well as the relative volume and flow of blood to the visualized area. Calculated results are displayed in the form of images or maps where each image represents the entire dynamic data set for that slice position.

The MTT map (Fig. **58–1C**) depicts the time required for fresh blood to completely replace that in the volume of interest. The time to peak (TTP) map is a simpler, related quantity that measures the arrival time of the bolus. Darker areas on the MTT map represent tissues having faster enhancement rates. In this example, normal gray matter (white asterisk) can be differentiated from normal white matter (black asterisk) due to intrinsic differences in MTT (in addition to demonstration of the pathologic findings previously discussed). The rCBV map (Fig. **58–1D**) is calculated based on changes in the intensity of pixels over time and conveys information regarding tissue blood volume within the displayed slice. Darker areas on this map correspond to regions with lower blood volume. Note that normal gray and white matter are well differentiated on the rCBV image due to the higher blood volume of gray matter. Relative cerebral blood flow maps (rCBF) (not shown) can also be calculated, but like MTT they require measurement of the signal intensity within an artery supplying the tissue of interest (the arterial input function).

59 Diffusion-Weighted Imaging

An early subacute left posterior cerebral artery (PCA) infarct is illustrated. Images were acquired with diffusion gradients applied in the x, y, and z directions and combined to form a single composite diffusion-weighted image (Fig. **59–1A**), also known as a trace-weighted image. Fig. **59–1B1–3** presents trace-weighted images with b-values of 500, 1000, and 0 (the latter thus simply an image with T2-weighting). The b-values are diffusion sensitivity factors. Increasing the b-value increases the conspicuity of the left PCA infarction relative to surrounding brain, but with a concomitant decrease in signal-to-noise ratio. A typical b-value for modern 1.5 T scanners is 1000 second/mm^2. Fig. **59–1B3** is an image acquired using the same pulse sequence, but without application of a diffusion gradient (b = 0). The high signal intensity of the infarct in this image reflects the T2 contribution, not diffusion. The apparent diffusion coefficient (ADC) map (Fig. **59–1B4**) is a calculated image, in which the effects of T1 and T2 have been removed. A lesion with restricted diffusion, such as an acute infarct, has high signal intensity (SI) on diffusion-weighted images, and low SI on the ADC map, the latter reflecting the low diffusion coefficient. Fluid-attenuated inversion recovery (FLAIR) (Fig. **59–1C**) and fast spin echo T2-weighted (Fig. **59–1D**) scans visualize the PCA infarct well, in this case, due to the presence of vasogenic edema (and thus a T2 change). Vasogenic edema only begins to occur sufficiently for detection by MR 8 hours after ictus. Thus, T2-weighted scans can miss very early infarcts.

Diffusion-weighted imaging (DWI) is a more sensitive means of detecting acute brain ischemia than conventional MR techniques or CT. Additional strong, pulsed gradients are applied on both sides of the 180° pulse in the three orthogonal axes using an echo planar type spin echo sequence. The time period between the application of these gradients is the diffusion observation period. The amplitude of the spin echo (signal) depends on the amount of water diffusion that occurs during this interval. In normal brain tissue, random water diffusion (Brownian motion) decreases the amplitude of the signal due to phase incoherence. With cytotoxic edema, there is no net change in water, only a change in its distribution. Within minutes following an ischemic insult, the amount of water within the intracellular compartment, where Brownian motion is restricted, increases. Phase coherence here is preserved and more signal recovered during the diffusion observation period, producing high SI. Note that although this is widely accepted as the theory behind acute stroke detection in diffusion-weighted MR, it has not been scientifically proven.

Hyperintensity on DWI, in and of itself, does not always correspond to a low diffusion value (as seen with cytotoxic edema, in the setting of acute infarction). Hyperintensity on DWI may be caused by "T2 shine through," with the change in signal intensity reflecting the T2, rather than diffusion, weighting of the image. To clarify the ambiguity inherent in DWI, an ADC map, in which there is no T2 contribution, is utilized. Acute (<24 hours) and early subacute (1 to 7 days) infarctions are hypointense on an ADC map (decreased diffusion) and hyperintense on DWI. Hyperacute (<6 hours) infarcts are also hyperintense on DWI (and hypointense on the ADC map), but isointense on T2-weighted scans (due to the presence of cytotoxic

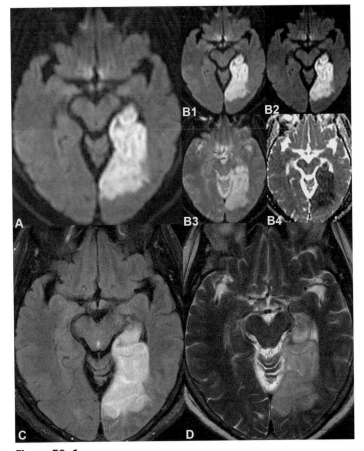

Figure 59–1

edema, without sufficient time for vasogenic edema to occur). After about a week (late subacute), normalization on DWI and ADC maps may be seen, with only T2 hyperintensity present as evidence of an interval infarct.

60 Diffusion Tensor Imaging

Slice-selective excitation and spatial encoding in MRI involves the switching of magnetic field gradients to temporarily create a spatial distribution of different resonance frequencies. Different resonance frequencies across a voxel cause a dephasing, which is commonly rephased with a matching gradient of opposite polarity or the same gradient prior to the 180° RF refocusing pulse. Let us consider for discussion purposes the frequency-encoding gradient. A dephasing gradient is applied of half the duration but the same amplitude prior to the 180° RF refocusing pulse. This provides an identical phase within all voxels at half the duration of the acquisition window. However, this is successful only if the magnetization within the voxel did not change location in the meantime. A change in location between switching of gradients causes a different phase history and thus insufficient rephasing. Insufficient rephasing results in diminished signal. This leads naturally to the topic of diffusion-weighted imaging (see case 59). A change in location can be based on diffusion. The effect of dephasing can be increased by using large gradient amplitudes of long durations with a long time duration between matching gradient pulses. Because these gradient pulses are employed simply for the visualization of diffusion, they are also called diffusion gradients. These gradient pulses have no effect on the signal from stationary tissue. Unfortunately, bulk motion, for example the expansion and contraction of the brain due to arterial pulsatile flow, contaminates any diffusion-weighted spin echo approach. The

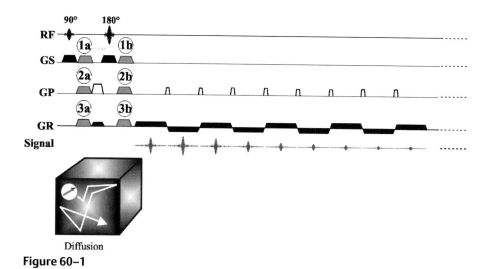

Diffusion

Figure 60–1

solution is to prepare the tissue using a spin echo and then rapidly read out the data using echo planar technique.

Fig. **60–1** presents the pulse diagram for a diffusion-weighted (spin echo) echo planar scan. A spin echo envelope is created using 90° and 180° RF pulses with matching "diffusion" gradients preceding and following the 180° RF pulse. The signal is read out using oscillating readout gradients. Phase encoding is performed, in this illustration, by "blipping" the phase encoding gradients during the ramp time of the readout gradients. Utilizing all six diffusion gradients (1a–3b) will lead to a quantifiable diffusion-weighted image. The diffusion is characterized by the apparent diffusion coefficient (ADC). MR can also provide information regarding the directional dependence of diffusion. For example, if only the diffusion gradients 1a and 1b are activated (Fig. **60–1**), only diffusion in the direction of slice selection will cause a hypointense appearance within the image. Repeating the scan with only 2a and 2b activated and again with only 3a and 3b activated provides directional information, in addition to magnitude information, regarding diffusion.

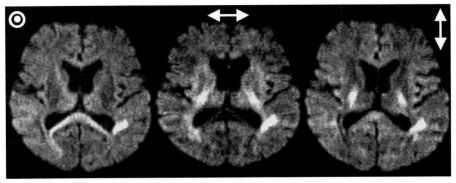

Figure 60–2

The directional dependence of diffusion is demonstrated in Fig. **60–2** (courtesy of A. Gregory Sorensen, MD, Massachusetts General Hospital, Boston). The arrows indicate the direction of the diffusion gradients. The axonal fiber bundles of the splenium of the corpus callosum have mainly a left to right direction. Diffusion anisotropy in white matter originates from its specific organization in bundles. Diffusion in the direction of the fibers is faster than in the perpendicular direction. Only molecular displacements that occur along the direction of the magnetic field gradients producing the diffusion weighting cause a visible change. With the diffusion weighting gradients applied perpendicular to the slice, the left to right and anterior to posterior displacement of water molecules within the splenium of the corpus callosum has no effect on image contrast. The splenium of the corpus callosum thus appears hyperintense. With the diffusion-weighting gradients applied left to right, the majority of molecular displacement within the splenium of the corpus callosum causes a dephasing, resulting in a hypointense appearance of the splenium of the corpus callosum.

A full description of molecular mobility along each direction including the correlation between the directions is given by the diffusion tensor. That diffusion tensor contains the information about direction and amount of diffusion in all directions. Seven measurements are necessary with different directions of diffusion weighting to calculate the diffusion tensor.

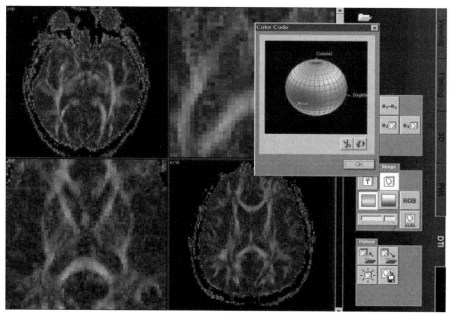

Figure 60–3   (see Color Plate 60–3, following page 130.)

Color maps have been suggested to display the amplitude and direction of diffusion (Fig. **60–3**). In this illustration, anisotropic diffusion derived from a diffusion tensor measurement is color encoded (courtesy of A. Gregory Sorensen, MD, Massachusetts General Hospital, Boston).

If the reference frame selected for the diffusion tensor is coincidentally along the principal direction of diffusion, the attenuation becomes a function of only the trace of the tensor. Turning and rotating the reference frame to the point where all off-diagonal terms of the diffusion tensor vanish allows the identification of the principal direction of diffusion within a single voxel.

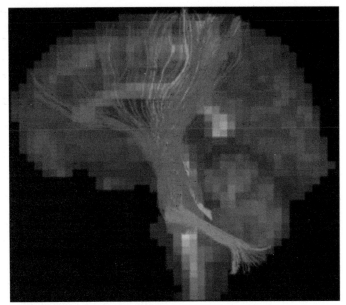

Figure 60–4   (see Color Plate 60–4, following page 130.)

Performing the same procedure for the adjacent voxel and connecting the diffusion vectors provides fiber orientation mapping (Fig. **60–4**, courtesy of David S. Tuch, PhD, Massachusetts General Hospital, Boston). Diffusion tensor imaging (DTI) has important potential clinical and research applications because it provides information about neuronal connectivity.

61 Blood Oxygen Level Dependent Imaging (BOLD): Theory

Blood oxygen level dependent imaging (BOLD), a type of functional MRI, involves the exploitation of the decrease in magnetic susceptibility caused by small changes in the volume of oxygenated blood to a specific region of the brain during and following increased neuronal activity. To understand the BOLD effect requires knowledge of the fundamental aspects of susceptibility imaging and the physiologic changes in the brain during activity. These concepts are discussed in this chapter.

Magnetic susceptibility (see case 93) relates to the ability of a material to become magnetized within an externally applied magnetic field and is measured by the magnetization of the material divided by the field strength. Materials with a strong magnetic susceptibility are referred to as ferromagnetic, those with a weak magnetic susceptibility are known as paramagnetic materials, and diamagnetic materials have little to no effect on the localized magnetic field with respect to surrounding tissues.

During an MRI examination, ferromagnetic and paramagnetic materials within the body take on magnetic characteristics causing localized changes or inhomogeneity within the field. Protons in the vicinity are affected by this change and experience a greater phase shift after a spin excitation, increasing T2* decay and leading to a reduction in localized signal. In the presence of strongly ferrous materials, a complete decay of signal occurs leading to a signal void in the image.

Hemoglobin, a constituent of red blood cells that carries oxygen, displays varying levels of susceptibility based on the amount of exposed iron found within its molecular structure. When oxygen is present, the iron in hemoglobin is shielded, reducing its magnetic susceptibility effect and leading to oxyhemoglobin being classified as diamagnetic. As oxygen is consumed, the exposed iron takes on magnetic properties leading to deoxyhemoglobin's paramagnetic effect. The presence of

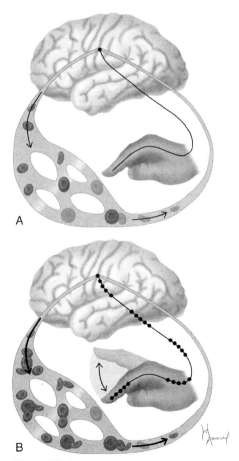

A

B

Figure 61–1

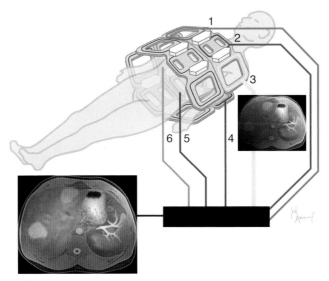

Color Plate 7-1   (see Figure 7-1, page 14.)

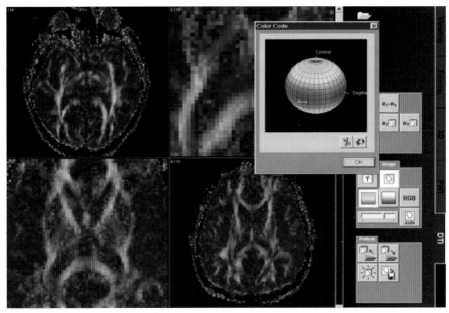

Color Plate 60-3   (see Figure 60-3, page 128.)

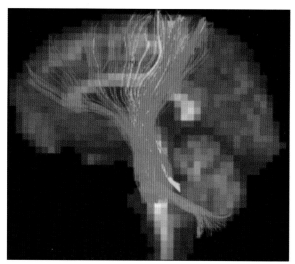

Color Plate 60-4 (see Figure 60-4, page 129.)

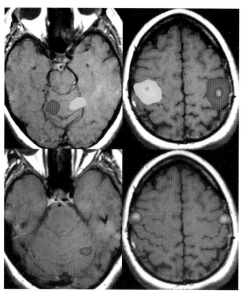

Color Plate 62-2 (see Figure 62-2, page 133.)

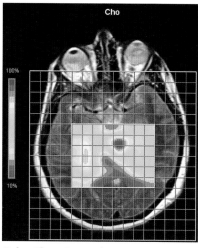

Color Plate 65-4 (see Figure 65-4, page 139.)

hemoglobin in both states throughout the microvasculature of the brain leads to a small, intrinsic level of magnetic susceptibility during MR examinations.

The activation of neurons during sensorimotor activity increases the consumption of oxygen within a specific area, decreasing the level of oxyhemoglobin. However, the reduced oxygen triggers adjacent capillaries to transport surplus levels of oxygenated blood to the area to facilitate further activity, increasing regional cerebral blood flow. The increased blood flow floods localized veins with oxyhemoglobin (Fig. **61–1**), leading to a small, localized decrease in susceptibility and increasing the MR signal. Both states, at rest (Fig. **61–1A**) and during activation (Fig. **61–1B**), are illustrated, with the activity in this example being finger tapping (for functional localization of primary motor cortex). With finger tapping, blood flow and oxygenated hemoglobin increases in the corresponding area of the motor cortex, leading to a signal change (albeit weak) that can be detected by MRI.

To visualize the subtle susceptibility change, sequences displaying a high level of sensitivity to magnetic susceptibility are used. Gradient echo based sequences, especially those used for echo planar imaging (EPI) (see case 39), use gradient polarity changes instead of RF pulses to rephase transverse magnetization and thus form an echo. This method leads to an increase in the viewable susceptibility changes by allowing the $T2^*$ effects to build up during the pulse sequence.

Higher field strengths (for example, 3 vs. 1.5 T) increase the effects of magnetic susceptibility and the visualization of the BOLD phenomenon. However, areas of strong susceptibility differences, such as air–tissue interfaces, induce distortion of the anatomy during EPI measurements. It is therefore important that the gradient hardware of MRI systems used to acquire BOLD data is efficient and powerful enough to produce high-quality images with limited geometric distortion.

62 Blood Oxygen Level Dependent Imaging (BOLD): Application

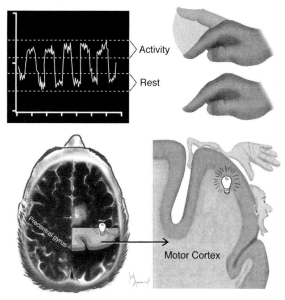

Figure 62–1

Changes in susceptibility induced by an increase in oxygenation within a localized area are very minute. To visualize the effect during an MRI measurement, the patient is asked to perform a series of tasks during the sequence acquisition to induce an alternating increase and decrease in the levels of oxyhemoglobin to a specific area of the sensory/motor cortex. For example, Fig. **62–1** illustrates finger tapping in a patient with an oligodendroglioma, World Health Organization (WHO) grade 2. The tumor lies just anterior to the precentral gyrus (primary motor area) in this instance.

The tasks are performed in a cycle called a paradigm specified in the sequence parameters prior to the sequence acquisition. The results are analyzed after completion of the examination. A statistical analysis (e.g., t-test, Z-score) is used to calculate the difference in the mean signal of the activation and rest portions of the echo planar imaging (EPI) measurement. The analysis assigns each pixel a level of significance based on the degree of real signal change. The results are then overlaid onto a T1- or T2-weighted image with the same field of view and slice coverage of the EPI measurement to provide the anatomic reference for analysis. Areas of distortion within the EPI measurement caused by stronger susceptibility influences at air–tissue interfaces in the sinuses can lead to an incorrect representation of the statistical results on the T1-weighted image. A gradient field map sequence showing areas of stronger susceptibility is often superimposed onto the combined T1 and mean image to show areas of possible distortion and misregistration.

Fig. **62–2A,B** displays the results of a bilateral finger tapping task paradigm displaying activation within the cerebral motor cortex as well as ipsilateral activation in the motor preparatory and timing area of the cerebellum. The gradient EPI sequence was programmed with a paradigm of 10 right followed by 10 left hand activations and performed over 60 measurements for a total scan time of approximately 3 minutes. The patient was instructed to touch the thumb to the fingers in a repeated series (e.g., 1-2-3-4-3-2-1) with 1 being the index finger and 4 being the fifth digit. The task

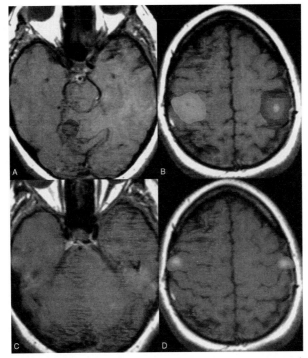

Figure 62–2 (see Color Plate 62–2, following page 130.)

was initiated with the start of the imaging sequence and began with the right hand for the first 10 and left hand for the second and so forth.

The second case (Fig. **62–2C,D**) involved an auditory paradigm where the patient was asked to repeat the word "seven" during the activation portion of the paradigm and remain silent during the rest portion. An alternation of 10 active and 10 inactive measurements was used and was performed for 100 measurements. Images for both examples were acquired at 3 T, with the higher field strength (as compared with 1.5 T) improving visualization of the BOLD effect.

Blood oxygen level dependent imaging has proven to be a valuable tool for analysis and mapping of the sensorimotor portion of the cerebral cortex, with ongoing research involving detailed aspects of thought and feelings and their effect on brain activity. (Images courtesy of Douglas H. Yock, MD, Abbott Northwestern Hospital, Minneapolis, MN.)

63 Proton Spectroscopy: Introduction

The displacement of normal anatomy due to mass lesions, the difference in molecular mobility affecting the relaxation times and thus image contrast, and finally the enhancement pattern following contrast administration are valuable diagnostic tools and mechanisms in MRI. In addition to imaging, MR offers the possibility to "visualize" the chemical environment via MR spectroscopy, examining the metabolism of areas in question **(Fig. 63–1)**. This information can be used to clarify ambiguous imaging findings.

The two common approaches in MR spectroscopy are single voxel spectroscopy (SVS) and chemical shift imaging (CSI). For SVS techniques the two main acquisition schemes are spin echo (SE) and stimulated echo acquisition method (STEAM).

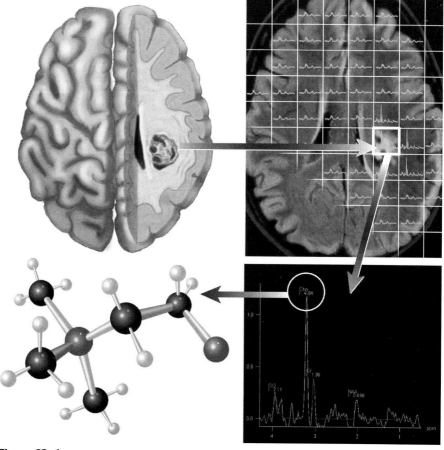

Figure 63–1

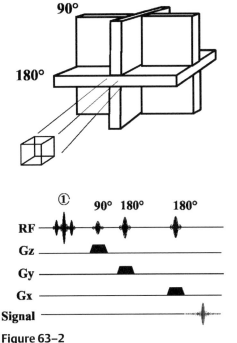

Figure 63–2

Fig. **63–2** illustrates the basic concept of SVS using a spin echo acquisition technique. The 90° pulse excites a slice. The slice-selective 180° pulse refocuses the transverse magnetization only in a row of tissue within the slice. A second 180° pulse then refocuses only the magnetization within a column of the row. Thus, only the signal originating in a single voxel remains. For proton spectroscopy, it is essential to suppress the water signal and, for regions outside the central nervous system, the lipid signal (1 in Fig. **63–2** marks the binomial RF pulse used to suppress either the water or lipid signal, see case 52).

Fig. **63–3** demonstrates the importance of suppressing the water signal. The metabolites of interest have a signal 100 times smaller than that of the water peak, and without water suppression would be poorly resolved.

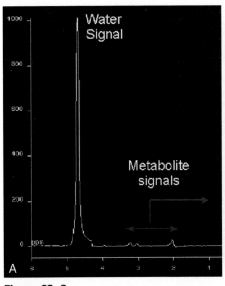
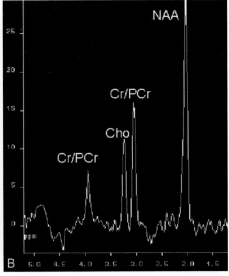

Figure 63–3

64 Proton Spectroscopy: SE Versus STEAM

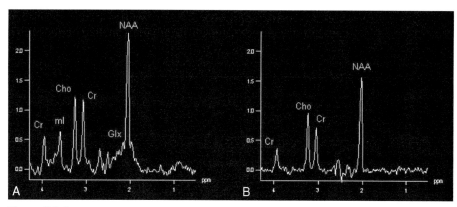

Figure 64-1

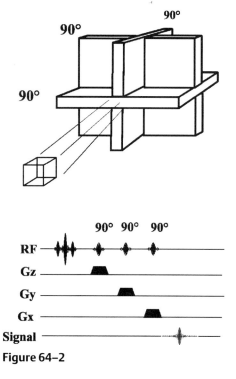

Figure 64-2

Fig. **64-1** demonstrates the effect of echo time in SE single voxel spectroscopy (SVS). Fig. **64-1A** was acquired with an echo time of 30 ms, whereas Fig. **64-1B** was acquired with an echo time of 144 ms. Variable TE values provide the ability to control the T2 "contrast" of the spectral peaks in the same way tissue T2 contrast is controlled in MRI. Short TE measurements are important for the detection of metabolite signals that have a short T2 decay and are not visible on long TE spectra.

The major healthy brain metabolite peaks that are seen on long TE spectra include *N*-acetylaspartate (NAA) at 2.02 ppm, choline (Cho) at 3.20 ppm, and creatine (Cr) at 3.02 ppm and 3.9 ppm. Short TE spectra contain additional peaks, which include *myo*-inositol (mI) at 3.56 ppm, glutamine and glutamate (Glx) between 2.05 to 2.5 ppm and 3.65 to 3.8 ppm, and glucose at 3.43 ppm.

Fig. **64-2** presents the pulse diagram for STEAM in SVS. There are three

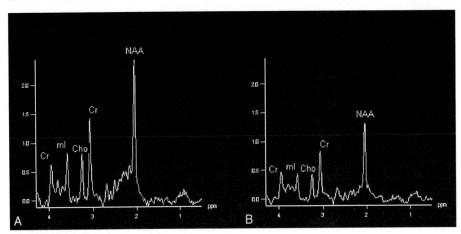

Figure 64–3

selective RF pulses applied in the presence of orthogonal magnetic field gradients (which specify the voxel of interest). Instead of one 90° and two 180° RF pulses, as in SE SVS, three 90° RF pulses are utilized. This excitation scheme creates stimulated echoes, rephasing ~50% of the original generated transverse magnetization. Although this means only half the SNR compared with SE SVS, the approach allows shorter echo times.

Fig. **64–3** presents a comparison between an SE SVS acquisition using an echo time of 30 ms (Fig. **64–3A**) and a STEAM SVS acquisition with an echo time of 20 ms (Fig. **64–3B**). STEAM SVS provides the same metabolic information as SE SVS and makes possible the use of a shorter TE, but produces only half the SNR of an SE SVS acquisition. SE SVS is less sensitive to spin motion. STEAM SVS is less demanding with respect to RF and is less sensitive to B_1 misadjustments.

65 Proton Spectroscopy: Chemical Shift Imaging

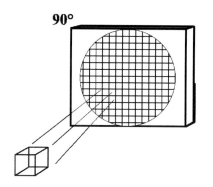

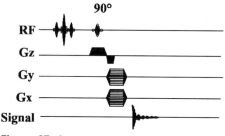

Figure 65–1

The frequency encoding gradient is omitted in localized spectroscopy, but the phase encoding gradient can be utilized, as in imaging, to encode spatial information into the signal. Fig. **65–1** is an illustration of a simple 2D chemical shift imaging (CSI) acquisition scheme sampling the free induction decay. A selective 90° RF pulse, in the presence of a magnetic field gradient, generates a transverse magnetization within the slice. Orthogonal magnetic field gradients of short duration encode spatial information into the signal to be acquired.

Fig. **65–2** illustrates the imaging setup for a 2D CSI acquisition. A single slice is defined through the area of interest, and then a box is specified within this (black lines). Spectra are then generated for all voxels within the box.

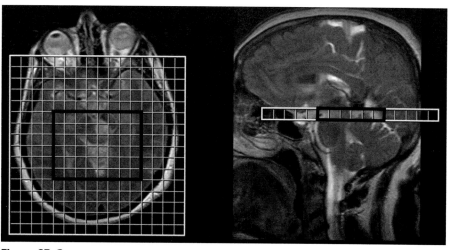

Figure 65–2

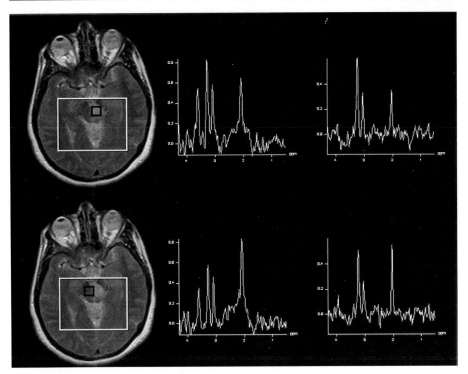

Figure 65–3

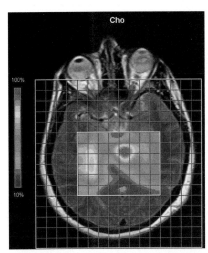

Figure 65–4 (see Color Plate 65–4, following page 130.)

Fig. **65–3** presents the spectra for a low-grade brainstem glioma. Data were acquired with a SE 2D CSI acquisition scheme, providing two spectra with echo times of 30 ms (second column) and 144 ms (third column). The first column shows the voxel corresponding to the spectra displayed on the same row. The first row spectra are from the lesion and the second row spectra from adjacent presumed normal brain. The lesion spectra demonstrate decreased NAA (a marker of neuronal integrity) and increased choline (a marker of myelin breakdown). The short TE spectrum demonstrates elevated *myo*-inositol (a marker of glial cells). Fig. **65–4** presents a color-coded choline metabolite map. (Images courtesy of Meng Law, MD, and Edmond A. Knopp, MD, New York University Medical Center, New York, New York.)

66 Number of Averages

The axial T2-weighted images of the cerebral peduncles and aqueduct (acquired using fast spin echo technique with a 2-mm slice thickness) presented in Fig. **66–1A–D** are from the same volunteer and were acquired using one, two, four, and eight averages, respectively. The number of averages is the number of times each line in k space is filled/sampled. This parameter is also known as the number of acquisitions, number of signals averaged (NSA), or number of excitations (NEX), depending on vendor. Because it represents the number of times each line in k space is filled, it directly affects scan time. In this example, the image in Fig. **66–1A** (1 NSA) was acquired in 32 seconds, in Fig. **66–1B** in 59 seconds, in Fig. **66–1C** in 1 minute 53 seconds, and in Fig. **66–1D** in 3 minutes 41 seconds (actual scan times). As the number of averages is increased, the voxels in each corresponding image have a higher signal-to-noise ratio (SNR), with each image thus progressively less "grainy" to the eye (from Fig. **66–1A** to Fig. **66–1D**).

The first and perhaps most important point to note is that doubling NSA doubles scan time but does not double SNR. Although scan time is linearly related to NSA, SNR is proportional to the square root of NSA (see case 12). Thus the scan time for Fig. **66–1B** is twice that of Fig. **66–1A**, yet the SNR of the image is only 41% (1.41 or the square root of two) higher. To double SNR using NSA, one would have to increase NSA, and therefore the overall scan time, by a factor of four. This is in stark contrast, for example, to doubling the slice thickness, which would increase SNR by a factor of two without an increase in scan time. This would result in the same increase in SNR as going from 1 NSA to 4 NSA (Fig. **66–1A** versus Fig. **66–1C**) without the resultant scan time increase. It is also important to note that one eventually reaches a point of diminishing returns in regard to the SNR increase provided by increasing NSA. With high SNR images, a further increase in SNR leads to little perceptible difference in the image or additional diagnostic information. For example, there is a marked improvement in image quality from Fig. **66–1A** to Fig. **66–1C**, but less perceptible change from a further doubling of NSA (and scan time) in Fig. **66–1D**.

Low-contrast lesion detectability, in particular, is improved by an increase in SNR. For example, in this comparison, the substantia nigra (with subtle low signal intensity, due to iron deposition) is best identified in the higher SNR images (arrows, Fig. **66–1D**). Averaging can also reduce the visual appearance of motion artifacts that originate from random or aperiodic motion. Using averaging in this way, however, has become less common in recent years as scan times for routine imaging became progressively shorter.

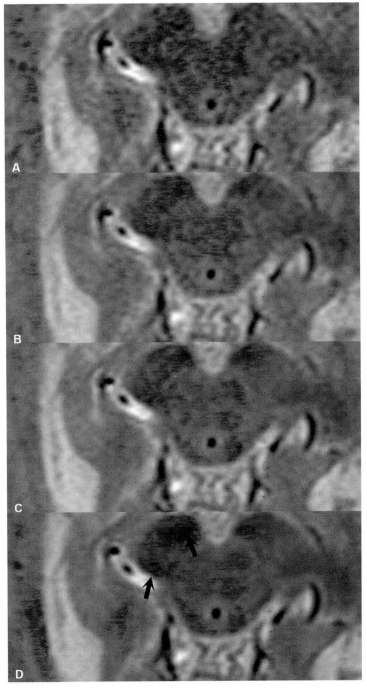

Figure 66–1

67 Slice Thickness

The thickness of an MR image, specified during scan setup, has a major impact on the quality of the resultant image, as well as on the imaging parameters used. When a thicker slice is acquired, the signal from more tissue is averaged, which can lead to poor anatomic definition and in particular to poorer definition of tissue interfaces. This phenomenon is known as volume averaging. The effect of volume averaging becomes especially problematic when the thickness of the acquired slice exceeds the size of a structure being evaluated. Therefore, it is desirable to acquire the thinnest slice possible to resolve structures with the greatest detail. However, as the slice thickness is reduced, the signal-to-noise ratio (SNR) is reduced by a proportional amount. To maintain adequate SNR (on thin slices) for definition of structures with low-contrast detectability, an increase in signal averaging, and thus time, must be applied.

Unfortunately, SNR is proportional to the *square root* of the number of averages, yet, as previously noted, *directly proportional* to slice thickness. Thus, halving the slice thickness reduces SNR by a factor of two. To compensate for this reduction, the number of averages has to be increased by a factor of four. Fig. **67–1A–C** presents images acquired with a slice thickness of 8, 4, and 2 mm, respectively. For these three scans, SNR was kept constant by changing the number of averages or excitations. Thus Fig. **67–1A** was acquired with one average, Fig. **67–1B** with four averages, and Fig. **67–1C** with 16 averages. This means that although Fig. **67–1C** shows a substantial increase in tissue contrast [note the improved delineation of cortical gray matter anteriorly and of the middle cerebral artery (MCA) branches within the sylvian fissure], the scan time for Fig. **67–1C** was 16 times that of Fig. **67–1A**. From a practical viewpoint, with certain scan sequences, very thin slices are simply not feasible due to the very long scan time that would be required. Fig. **67–1D** demonstrates a slice thickness reduction from 8 to 2 mm without an increase in averaging to compensate for the loss in SNR. The result is a very "noisy" or low SNR image. This has little effect on high-contrast structures such as the flow voids from MCA branch vessels (black arrows) traveling through the slice, but an appreciable effect on low contrast structures such as the putamen, globus pallidus, caudate nucleus, and especially the gray-white matter differentiation (white arrow). When selecting the thickness of slices to be acquired, scan time, slice coverage, SNR, and (high and low) contrast detectability must all be taken into consideration.

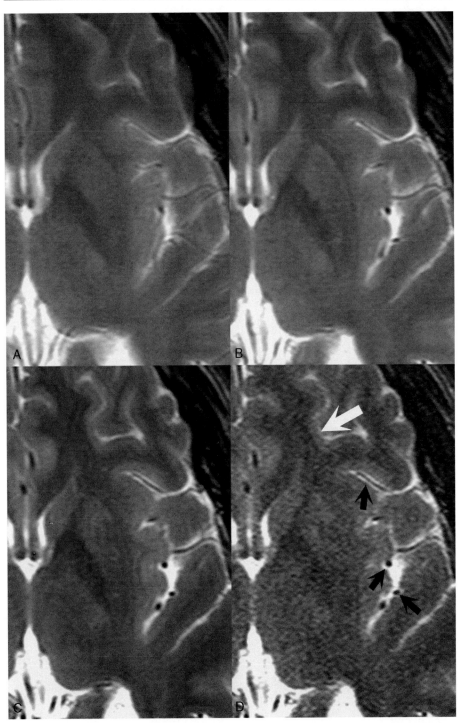

Figure 67–1

68 Slice Profile

Ideally, a slice in MRI should experience a uniform radiofrequency (RF) excitation throughout its thickness. Sharp, distinct edges should exist with no excitation extending beyond slice boundaries. However, in practice the spatial excitation of spins is invariably a distribution ranging from the RF flip angle specified at the center of the

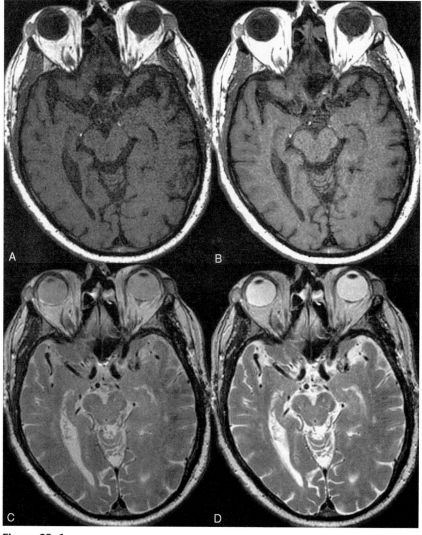

Figure 68–1

slice to largely reduced flip angles at the ill-defined edges that excite regions well beyond the desired thickness. The resultant change in signal across the thickness of a slice is termed the slice profile.

Thus, in multislice imaging (the mainstay of clinical MR today), a slice of interest may suffer interference, or "crosstalk," from neighboring slices caused by RF excitation that extends beyond their slice boundaries. Signal-to-noise ratio (SNR) loss (compare Fig. **68–1A**, which was performed with no gap, with Fig. **68–1B**, which was performed with a 100% gap) and contrast changes (compare Fig. **68–1C**, which was performed with no gap, with Fig. **68–1D**, which was performed with a 100% gap) within each slice may result. When the gap between slices is reduced, slice-to-slice interference becomes more likely. True contiguity is theoretically not possible in two-dimensional multislice MRI, with the worst effects seen at 0% slice gaps where interference among slices is the greatest. Conversely, the best results occur when the gap is large enough so that neighboring slice excitations do not interfere with each other. Gaps of 10% to 30% are common in current clinical practice.

Because of slice profiles, a lesion directly in the center (width-wise) of a slice is seen best (lesion 'A' in Fig. **68–2**), and a lesion near the edge (lesion 'B' in Fig. **68–2**) potentially less well [**Fig. 68–2** shows fluid-attenuated inversion recovery (FLAIR) imaging in multiple sclerosis]. This also means that small lesions can be missed in between slices, thus one reason for imaging in two planes in disease processes such as multiple sclerosis and (postcontrast) brain metastases.

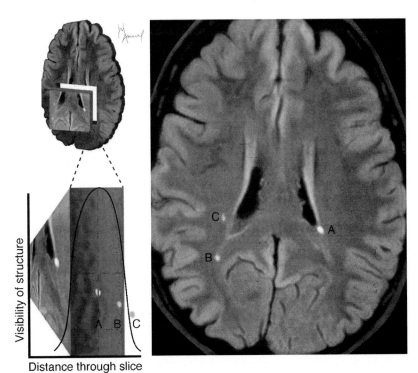

Figure 68–2

69 Slice Excitation Order (in Fast Spin Echo Imaging)

In MRI, an ideal RF pulse is uniform across the slice thickness, with sharp, distinct edges and no excitation extending beyond slice boundaries. In practice however, the spatial excitation of spins is invariably a distribution ranging from the correct RF excitation flip angle at the center of the slice to largely reduced flip angles at the ill-defined edges (see case 68). This results in partial excitation of regions in the neighborhood of the excited slice, but beyond its theoretical edge. Time-limited RF pulses are inherently imperfect, resulting in nonrectangular slice profiles. In multislice fast spin echo imaging, the situation is especially critical, because the slice profile is defined by the overlapping RF profiles of the excitation pulse as well as of all the 180° refocusing pulses applied over the duration of the echo train. In Fig. **69–1**, *1* shows the overlapping RF profiles that result due to the acquisition of multiple echoes (each with different phase encoding) that is the basis for fast spin echo technique; and *2* depicts sequential slice acquisition using a fast spin echo sequence. The nonideal RF profiles of the 90° excitation pulse as well as those of the 180° RF refocusing pulses result in a decrease in the available longitudinal magnetization in the adjacent slices. To minimize this influence, an interleaved acquisition (*3* in Fig. **69–1**) may be performed by chronologically altering the order in which slices are excited. The first, third, fifth, and subsequent slices are excited in sequence, followed then by the second, fourth, sixth, and subsequent slices. In this way, the longitudinal magnetization

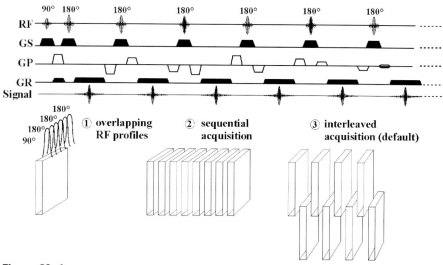

Figure 69–1

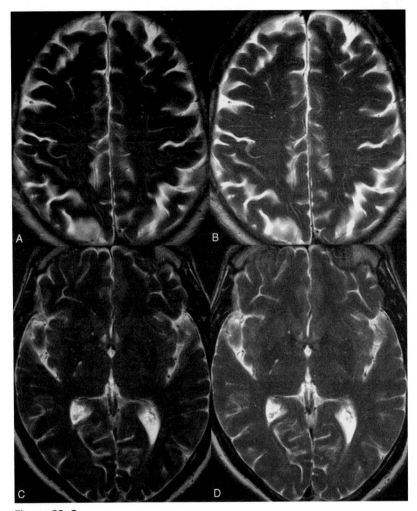

Figure 69–2

within adjacent slices has additional time for recovery, during the time between acquisition of the data for the other slice group and application of the next RF excitation and refocusing pulses.

Fig. **69–2A–D** presents two fast spin echo multislice acquisitions, with images acquired sequentially (**A,C**) and in an interleaved fashion (**B,D**). The differences are not due to windowing (note that fat has a similar appearance on both scans). Saturation effects due to overlapping excitation and refocusing profiles (between adjacent slices) lead to an overall signal loss, which is accentuated with sequential acquisition. Note the markedly lower SNR of normal brain in **A** and **C** as compared with **B** and **D**, despite the fact that both scans were acquired using the same imaging parameters.

70 Slice Orientation

One of the major advantages of MR is the ability to acquire thin slices at any angle or orientation within the body through the use of gradient and RF hardware. Nuclei subjected to a homogeneous, static magnetic field resonate with a frequency related to that field. At 1.5 T, the frequency for hydrogen (^{1}H) is ~63 MHz. An RF pulse generated at this specific frequency causes all the resonating hydrogen nuclei within the homogeneous field to absorb and release energy, making spatial localization of a specific tissue impossible. However, when a magnetic field gradient is applied, the nuclei experience different magnetic field strengths and begin to resonate at different frequencies based on their position. An RF pulse can thus be tuned to a specific frequency to excite only nuclei in a desired location based on their resonant frequency. This is the concept that makes slices in any orientation possible.

MRI systems are equipped with three spatial encoding gradients (x, y, and z) made of loops of wire that either add to or subtract from the main magnetic field when a current is passed through them. A gradient change induced in only one direction results in the ability to create a slice orthogonal to the gradient. Therefore, turning on the gradient in the x direction results in sagittal slices, y in coronal slices, and z (along the bore of the magnet) in transverse (axial) slices. The thickness of a slice can be defined by either adjusting the bandwidth of the RF pulse to increase or decrease the range of frequencies included and therefore protons excited by the pulse, or by increasing or decreasing the strength of the gradient. Fig. **70–1** demonstrates the effect that turning on the z gradient would have on the magnetic field and resulting resonant frequency across the field of view. An RF pulse deposited at a specific frequency (e.g., 64 MHz) would excite only those protons (in this example, an axial slice through the ankles) making spatial localization of a specific location and slice selection possible. Gradient changes made in multiple directions (e.g., z and y) allow slices to be tilted away from a single axis.

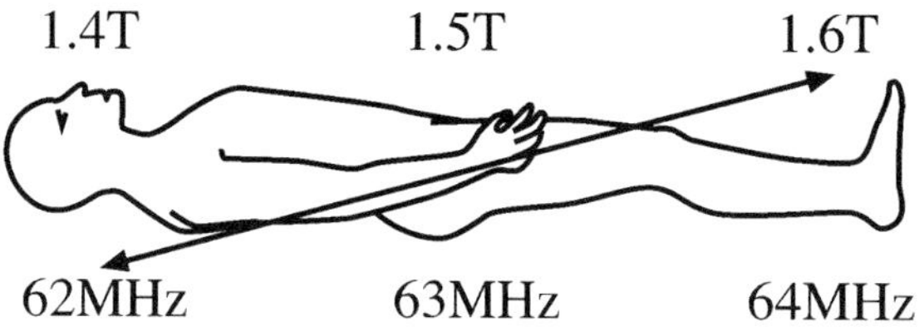

1.4T   1.5T   1.6T

62MHz   63MHz   64MHz

Figure 70–1

Fig. **70–2A** demonstrates axial slices rotated into the coronal plane positioned on a midsagittal T2-weighted image of the lumbar spine, with Fig. **70–2B** illustrating one of the resulting images from this specified coronal block of slices. Fig. **70–3A** again depicts the sagittal image acquired for slice positioning, with a tilted coronal block of

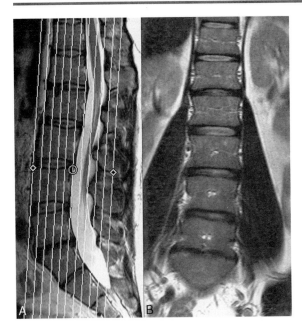

Figure 70–2

slices now specified for imaging of the sacrum. The sacrum and its neural foramina are in particular well evaluated on such a tilted coronal image (Fig. **70–3B**), with clinical application for imaging of sacral insufficiency fractures and perineural (Tarlov) cysts.

Lumbar spine imaging takes particular advantage of the ability to tilt slices in MRI, with two different approaches used for axial imaging. In some clinics, individual blocks of images (all part of a single axial acquisition) are tilted to the individual disk spaces being examined, whereas in others a single block of images is acquired tilted to match the orientation of one level. Difficulty in patient positioning can be corrected by tilting the images acquired, for example by the use of a coronal scout with subsequent correction of the sagittal scan setup so that true sagittal images are acquired (depicting the spinal canal in its entirety on one image). Cardiac imaging routinely employs double oblique images, once again made possible by use of the gradients.

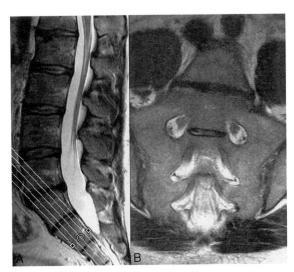

Figure 70–3

71 Field of View (FOV)

The field of view (FOV) is defined as the dimensions of the exact anatomic region included in a scan. In MR, the FOV may be square or asymmetric. Depending on the vendor, it is specified in millimeters or centimeters. The FOV is also the mathematical product of the acquisition matrix and the pixel dimensions. For example, if 512 readout and 256 phase encoding steps are specified in a scan for which the pixel dimensions are chosen to be 0.45 × 0.9 mm, the FOV would be 512 × 0.45 mm = 230 mm by 256 × 0.9 mm = 230 mm (and thus in this instance a square FOV, despite the use of a rectangular pixel). Head imaging is typically performed today with a FOV of 230 mm or less, to achieve high in-plane spatial resolution. Depending on body habitus, the FOV for a scan of the upper abdomen may be as large as 400 mm.

The choice of FOV in clinical work is somewhat complex, involving a trade-off between the signal-to-noise ratio (SNR) and spatial resolution, and depending as well on the size of the body part being scanned. Frequently a smaller FOV is desired for the improved spatial resolution it affords. However, SNR is proportional to the square of the FOV (because the FOV specifies both dimensions of a pixel and thus its area), assuming the image matrix is held constant. If the FOV is halved, SNR decreases by a factor of four. Less drastic changes are the norm in clinical imaging. If the resolution in a particular scan is slightly less than desired, and SNR is not a limiting factor, then a slight reduction in FOV may be worthwhile. For example, a 20% smaller FOV provides 20% better resolution in both pixel dimensions, at the expense of a 40% reduction in SNR:

$$SNR \propto FOV(r) \times FOV(p)$$
where FOV(r) and FOV(p) are the FOV in the readout and phase encoding directions, respectively

The T2-weighted images presented differ only in the choice of FOV, which was 350 vs. 250 vs. 150 mm (Fig. **71–1A–C**). The visual magnification of the images was held constant for Fig. **71–1A–C**. One immediate problem with using a very small FOV becomes evident in Fig. **71–1C**—the wraparound of the scalp from one side onto the other (arrow). Fig. **71–1D** compares the image in Fig. **71–1A** and that in Fig. **71–1C**, visually magnifying **A** to match anatomically **C**. The decrease in SNR in Fig. **71–1C** is reflected by the graininess of the image; however, the increased spatial resolution improves anatomic depiction of small structures such as a vessel within a sulcus (black arrow) and a small dilated perivascular space (white arrow). In patients with exceptionally large heads, employing the usual FOV can lead to wraparound, particularly in the sagittal plane, with the nose (or jaw) overlapping the posterior part of the head. Wraparound (aliasing) artifact is caused by undersampling. To eliminate wraparound, oversampling can be employed in the readout (frequency encoding) dimension at no cost in scan time or SNR. Oversampling in the phase encoding direction leads to increased scan time (but improved SNR) and is less commonly used. The choice of direction for the readout gradient is thus often determined by the anatomic part and

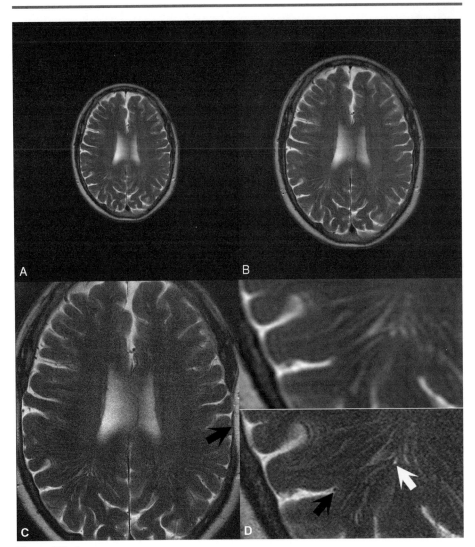

Figure 71–1

the possibility of aliasing, for example with the readout direction chosen routinely to be craniocaudal in coronal imaging of the head to eliminate wraparound from the neck.

72 Field of View: Rectangular

The field of view (FOV) defines the part of the patient to be imaged. This is chosen prior to scan acquisition, and need not be square. Indeed, under certain circumstances a reduced FOV along one axis can be advantageous. The topic of this case is the choice of the FOV in the phase encoding direction.

In Fig. **72–1**, the FOV in the phase encoding direction (right to left in this instance) was changed from 100% (Fig. **72–1A**) to 75% (Fig. **72–1B**) to 50% (Fig. **72–1C**). Images are displayed as acquired, without cropping or differential magnification. Because the pixel size was held constant, fewer phase encoding steps were required for Fig. **72–1B** (three-fourths the number) and Fig. **72–1C** (one-half the number). Scan time is directly proportional to the number of phase encoding steps, and so the scan time of Fig. **72–1B** was three-fourths that of Fig. **72–1A**, and that for Fig. **72–1C** one-half that of Fig. **72–1A**. However, as illustrated, there are two potential problems associated with using this approach, also termed a "rectangular" FOV. The first problem is the wraparound (aliasing) artifact. If the part of the patient being scanned extends beyond the FOV in the phase encoding direction, it will appear superimposed on top of the image on the other side. Thus in Fig. **72–1C** the right part of the head appears superimposed over the (anatomic) left side of the image, and the left part of the head over the right side of the image (arrows). The second problem is reduced SNR. Using fewer phase encoding steps (p) leads to lower SNR (SNR $\propto \sqrt{p}$). SNR decreased from (a relative value of) 1 in Fig. **72–1A** to 0.87 in Fig. **72–1B** to 0.71 in Fig. **72–1C**. In Fig. **72–1D**, the FOV has been kept the same as in Fig. **72–1C** but the number of acquisitions (averages) doubled. This counters the decrease in SNR due to the choice of FOV. Thus, the SNR in Fig. **72–1A** and Fig. **72–1D** are the same, as are the scan time and pixel size.

Fig. **72–1E,F** compares similarly magnified parts of Fig. **72–1C** (top) to Fig. **72–1D** (bottom), to illustrate better the SNR loss, The subtle graininess of the image on the top (Fig. **72–1E**) is due to its lower SNR. Note that if the area of interest is near to the center of the FOV, then some image wrap can be tolerated. Very little image artifact is noted in these closely cropped images.

A rectangular FOV is commonly used in axial head imaging (without changing the number of averages), decreasing scan time with only a minimal reduction in SNR. Fig. **72–1B** is an example of this application, with the FOV in the phase encoding direction chosen to closely match the dimension of the head (right to left). A rectangular FOV finds similar application in imaging of other body parts that have a reduced width in one dimension (such as the wrist on axial imaging). It should be noted that in the preceding discussion the pixel size has been assumed to be square. This need not be the case, and the shape of the pixel can be varied together with the FOV, thus also influencing spatial resolution along one axis. With modern MR scanners, the increment by which the FOV, the number of phase encoding steps, and the number of readout steps can be changed is almost unlimited.

In reference to aliasing, with the scanners delivered today, this phenomenon is restricted to the phase encoding direction. Aliasing in the readout or frequency encoding direction, although a problem in the past (and countered by oversampling), is no longer an issue.

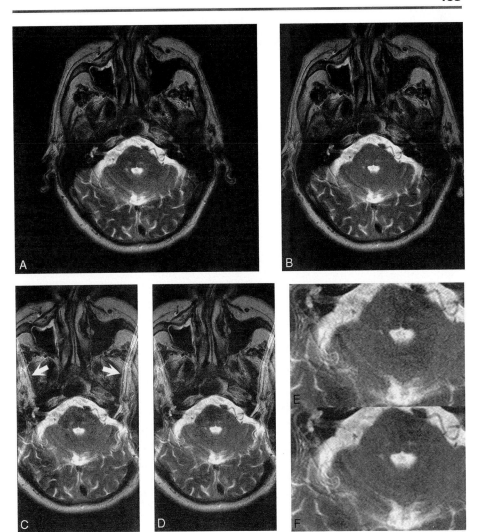

Figure 72–1

73 Matrix Size: Read

The images presented demonstrate the effect of changing the acquisition matrix in the frequency encoding (readout) direction. All are T2-weighted fast spin echo sagittal images of the lumbar spine. The acquisition matrix (readout × phase encoding) was 1024 × 256 for Fig. **73–1A**, 512 × 256 for Fig. **73–1B**, and 256 × 256 for both Fig. **73–2A** and Fig. **73–2B**. The image in Fig. **73–2B** was further interpolated to 512 × 512 prior to display.

When the MR signal (echo) is produced it is sampled in the presence of a gradient magnetic field. This gradient is thus referred to as the "readout" or "read" gradient. The digital sampling (encoding) of the echo produces data points along the frequency direction of k space. The number of samples taken during the readout period is determined by the desired number of pixels in the frequency encoding direction. Not to confuse the issue, but this is why one may see the read gradient referred to as the "frequency encoding" gradient. If a frequency resolution of 512 pixels is desired, then

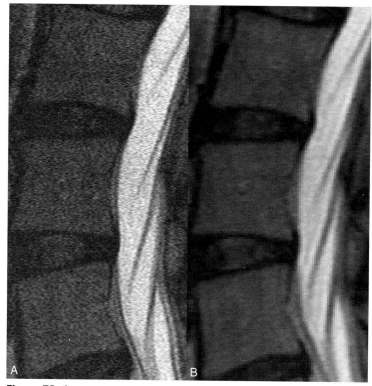

Figure 73–1

the echo will be sampled 512 times during the readout period (Fig. **73–1B**). Increasing the frequency resolution to 1024 results in 1024 samples taken during readout (Fig. **73–1A**). In most clinical imaging situations, the frequency acquisition matrix is equal to or greater than the phase matrix, because the frequency matrix does not affect scan time.

Although increasing the acquisition matrix in the read direction does not affect scan time, it does affect the signal-to-noise ratio (SNR) of the image. As the pixel size is reduced, the MR signal is reduced, making the noise more obvious (leading to the "grainy" appearance of the image). One can easily see that Fig. **73–1A** (1024 × 256) has higher spatial resolution but also much lower SNR than Fig. **73–1B** (512 × 256). Reducing the read matrix further to 256 (Fig. **73–2A,B**) increases SNR again, but results in even lower spatial resolution.

MR images are commonly interpolated to higher matrices for display purposes. This interpolation, however, merely "smooths" out the pixels one would see in the image if it were not interpolated (compare Fig. **73–2A** and **B**). The degree of interpolation and the algorithm used depend on the MR system vendor. Note that the acquisition matrix, not the reconstructed or displayed matrix, determines the spatial resolution of an MR image.

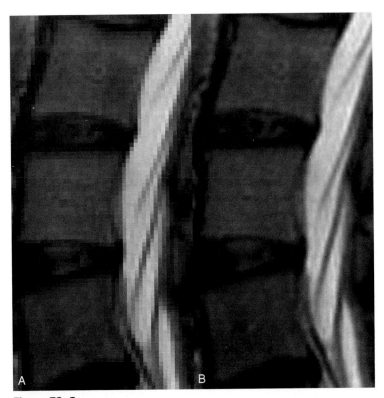

Figure 73–2

74 Matrix Size: Phase

Fig. **74–1A,B** presents sagittal T2-weighted images of the midlumbar spine demonstrating mild degenerative disk disease. Fig. **74–2A,B** presents sagittal T1-weighted images, in a different patient, of the lower thoracic and upper lumbar spine at the level of the conus medullaris, revealing a benign chronic compression fracture of L1.

The choice of phase encoding matrix determines the number of pixels along the phase encoding direction of the acquired FOV. This determines how many different lines of k space will be filled during the acquisition. Thus the number of phase encoding steps directly effects scan time. Flow and/or motion artifacts also are propagated along the phase encoding direction. Additionally, assuming the display and acquired FOV are identical, if there is significant signal from excited tissue outside the FOV, it will wrap, or fold over, into the displayed FOV (see case 102). This occurs in both the phase and frequency direction and is overcome by oversampling. Oversampling increases the scan time when applied in the phase encoding direction (except for single shot techniques), assuming that all other parameters and in particular the number of signals averaged are held constant.

Fig. **74–1A** was acquired using a 256 read matrix and 128 phase matrix. Fig. **74–1B** was acquired with a 256 read and 256 phase matrix. The phase encoding direction in both examples was in the craniocaudal direction, with 100% oversampling. The scan time for Fig. **74–1A** was 2:08 and for Fig. **74–1B** 4:08. Although the scan time for Fig. **74–1B** was twice that of Fig. **74–1A**, with an acquired FOV of 280 mm the

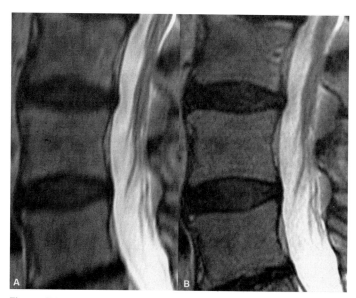

Figure 74–1

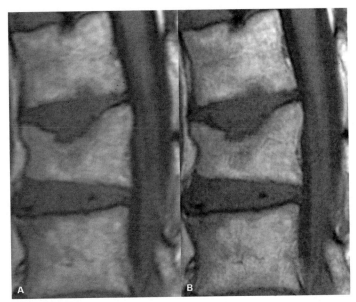

Figure 74–2

pixel dimension in the phase direction for Fig. **74–1A** was 2.2 mm and that for Fig. **74–1B** 1.1 mm. Fig. **74–1B** thus has higher spatial resolution. As an aside, it is worthwhile noting that selecting the phase direction to be craniocaudal for sagittal T2-weighted fast spin echo (FSE) imaging of the spine can substantially reduce the conspicuity of CSF pulsation artifacts.

The image in Fig. **74–2A** was acquired using a read matrix of 512 and a phase matrix of 256. Fig. **74–2B** was acquired using a read matrix of 512 and a phase matrix of 512. The scan time for Fig. **74–2A** was 3:38 and that for Fig. **74–2B** 7:15. With the higher matrix size, the pixel dimension in Fig. **74–2B** in the phase encoding direction is reduced and spatial resolution increased. The pixel dimension in the phase (and read) direction for Fig. **74–2B** is just over 0.5 mm. One will also note that as the pixel size is reduced, SNR is reduced, with the result being an increase in the overall "grainy" appearance of the image. However, one should recall that with pixel size constant, increasing the phase encoding matrix actually increases SNR (with SNR $\propto \sqrt{[\text{number of phase encoding steps}]}$).

In summary, spatial resolution can be improved by increasing the number of phase encoding steps, which results in a smaller pixel dimension along the phase FOV. However, because this increases the number of k-space lines acquired, it also increases scan time. Reducing the pixel size, however, in either the read or phase direction, reduces SNR, assuming all other parameters are held constant.

75 Partial Fourier

Fig. **75–1A** and Fig. **75–1B** represent half-Fourier and conventional Fourier techniques, respectively, of a T1-weighted image. The image in Fig. **75–1A** was acquired in approximately half the time as the image in Fig. **75–1B**. This is because in partial Fourier, only a fraction of the phase encoding steps are sampled (Fig. **75–1C**, the image data in k space corresponding to Fig. **75–1A**), whereas in conventional Fourier, all

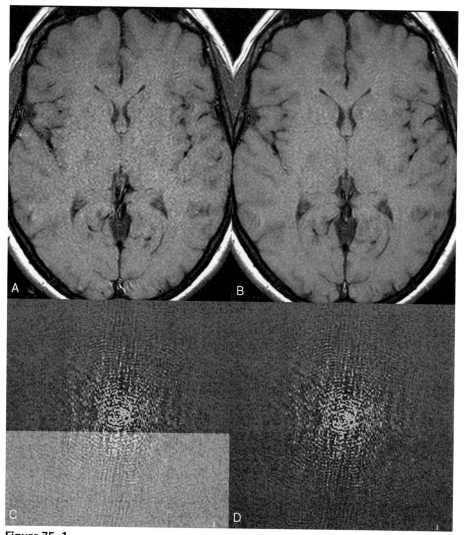

Figure 75–1

phase encoding steps are incorporated into the final image (Fig. **75–1D**). Spatial resolution is preserved between the two images, that is, there is equal demarcation between adjacent structures of differing signal intensity with either technique. However, there is a resultant decrease in signal-to-noise ratio (SNR) (see case 74), which accounts for the "noisier" image seen in Fig. **75–1A**.

Fourier transform analysis is the process by which MR signals in the form of k space are transformed into pixel data of the final image. Specifically, this involves converting data in terms of the time domain (k space) to data in terms of the frequency domain (image). Fourier analysis may occur via single or multidimensional techniques.

As discussed earlier, in k space (see case 10) the vertical and horizontal axes represent phase encoding and frequency encoding, respectively (see cases 73 and 74). In a 256×256 (readout $\times$ phase-encoding) matrix, therefore, 256 phase encoding steps occur from position -127 to 128. It is not absolutely necessary to obtain the entire data set from -127 to 128 because there is a type of mathematical symmetry (conjugate symmetry) that exists between -127 to 0 and 1 to 128. Therefore, data from a fraction (at least half) of k space may be used to create the entire image. This process is termed partial Fourier technique. In standard practice, the size of the measured matrix may range from half to all in some given increment (e.g., four eighths, five eighths, etc.). Of note is that in half-Fourier, slightly more than 50% of the phase encoding steps are measured so as to ensure adequate data incorporation of the center of k space. The true benefit of partial Fourier technique is a percentage decrease in acquisition time by a factor equal to the percentage decrease in the number of measured phase encoding steps. With all other imaging parameters remaining constant, partial Fourier technique preserves spatial resolution (see case 11). This technique, however, decreases SNR due to a decrease in the total number of phase encoding steps. This reflects a loss of redundant data and thus increases the relative impact of error (noise) on the final image. In half-Fourier technique, for example, acquisition time is approximately halved with a decrease in SNR by a factor of 1.4. Note, however, that partial Fourier does not reduce scan times in fast spin echo due to the manner in which data are acquired with such scan techniques.

With a decrease in SNR from a fewer number of sampled phase encoding steps, there is a predictable decrease in the visualization of low-contrast lesions (i.e., multiple sclerosis plaques). However, because spatial resolution is preserved, partial Fourier has clinical utility for high-contrast objects (i.e., large tumors in T2-weighted scans). Thus, partial Fourier techniques must be used with discretion.

76 Image Interpolation (Zero Filling)

A common display size on a monitor is a 512 × 512 pixel matrix. The image acquisition matrix in MRI is often lower, and some interpolation may be performed automatically. A straightforward approach is to place an empty pixel between pixels (step 1 in Fig.

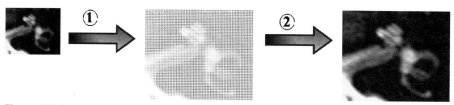

Figure 76–1

76–1) and assign the amplitude of this pixel to be the average value of the adjacent pixels (linear interpolation, step 2 in Fig. **76–1**). A more advanced solution is the use of a bicubic spline interpolation. In this case the value of not only the adjacent pixel is taken into account, but also that of the following pixel. The result is smoother, masking the truly measured spatial resolution. For Fourier encoding, a low spatial resolution matrix corresponds to a small k space. In any k-space matrix, the outer data points contain the signal for the magnetization of adjacent voxels having opposite signs. Consider a homogeneous phantom that fills the entire field of view, the opposing adjacent magnetizations will induce no signal, resulting in zero values for those data points. Doubling the raw data matrix size and filling the missing data points with the value zero will not improve the spatial resolution, but will mimic the measurement of a higher resolution matrix. Zero filling corresponds to a voxel-shifted interpolation and reduces the partial volume effects of the pixel grid used for reconstruction. Fig. **76–2**

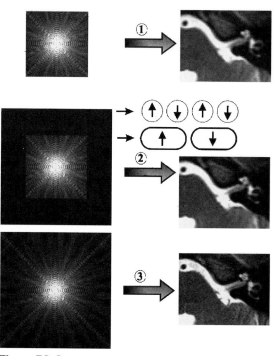

Figure 76–2

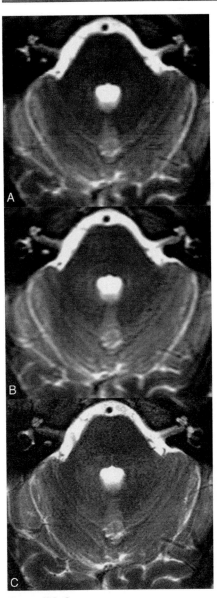

Figure 76–3

illustrates Fourier interpolation as applied in MRI. In step 1, the k-space data and corresponding image for a 128 × 128 acquisition matrix is illustrated. In step 2, zero filling is used to expand k space. The resulting interpolated 256 × 256 image is compared with a true 256 × 256 acquisition in step 3. In Fig. **76–3**, a T2-weighted axial image of the brain at the level of the pons acquired using a 256 × 256 matrix (Fig. **76–3A**) is compared with the same image interpolated to 512 × 512 using zero filling in k space (Fig. **76–3B**) and a true 512 × 512 acquisition (Fig. **76–3C**).

In the case of small structures, for example, a small vessel in a time-of-flight MRA of a size close to the spatial resolution of the measurement, the intensity of the representing pixel depends on where the vessel is located relative to the measurement grid. If the vessel is within a single voxel, the signal will be very bright. If the vessel lies between two voxels, these two voxels will share the intensity, resulting in a less dominant vessel appearance. Theoretically, the appearance will be improved by shifting the measurement grid, which is identical to a voxel shift, eliminating the above mentioned partial volume effect. Zero filling in k space corresponds to a voxel shift. In other words, spatial resolution is not improved, but the partial volume artifacts are significantly reduced.

77 Phase Images

Phase images are commonly used in MR flow quantification. As explained previously, phase describes the position of the transverse magnetization within the transverse plane. Magnetic field gradients are used during slice-selective excitation and for the purpose of spatial encoding. Any magnetic field gradient gives rise to a variation in resonance frequencies across the object. This results in a different phase position for the transverse magnetizations within the voxel in the direction of the field gradient. In some cases, this is undesirable and a compensating field gradient is applied after the slice selection (GS) or before the readout (GR) gradient. However, this rephasing will be successful only if the voxel within the object does not move between, or during, switching of the field gradients. If motion does occur, the phase history of the transverse magnetizations will be different, resulting in incomplete rephasing. Fig. **77–1** presents the pulse diagram of a flow quantification or phase contrast acquisition scheme. Two sequences, one flow compensated and the other flow sensitized, are usually executed in an interleaved fashion. For tissues or fluids moving with a constant velocity, a three-lobe gradient structure will ensure that the phase is null at the echo for both moving and stationary tissue (*1* in Fig. **77–1**). Such a sequence is termed flow-insensitive or flow-compensated (see case 99). "Detuning" the gradient arrangement (as indicated by *2* in Fig. **77–1**) for the slice-selective gradient (GS) results in through-plane "flow-sensitivity." The transverse magnetization within fluids that are moving will have a different phase position (*2* in Fig. **77–1**) compared with that measured with flow compensation (*1* in Fig. **77–1**). The difference in phase, $\Delta\phi$, is directly proportional to the velocity of the flow and can be used for quantification. The magnitude of the "vector" ΔM between the two transverse magnetizations (*1* and *2* in Fig. **77–1**) is used in phase-contrast MR angiography (PC-MRA).

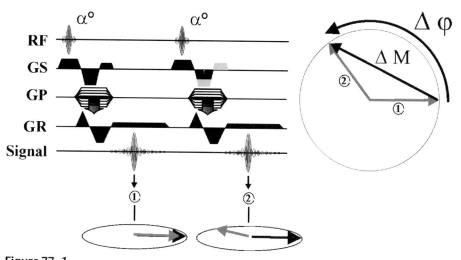

Figure 77–1

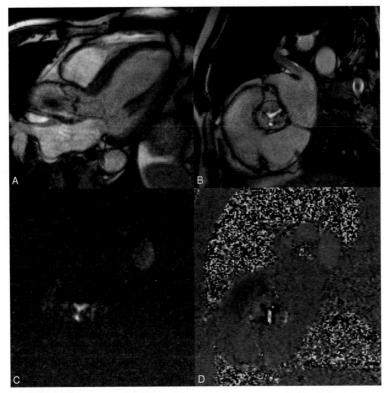

Figure 77–2

Fig. **77–2** presents images of a patient with severe aortic insufficiency (regurgitation). Fig. **77–2A** and **B** present images (with the valve in cross section and in plane) acquired utilizing true fast imaging with steady-state precession (trueFISP). Flow-sensitive sequences are used to evaluate the severity of the stenosis. Fig. **77–2C** is the magnitude image ΔM of the flow-sensitive acquisition, corresponding in anatomic position to Fig. **77–2B**. Note that the phase images Δφ of the flow-sensitized acquisition (Fig. **77–2D**) indicate not only the magnitude but also the direction of flow. Flow toward the observer is hyperintense, flow away from the observer is hypointense. If the phase change exceeds 180° (π), hypointense and hyperintense voxels will be observed in the same vessel, as in this case, indicating that the selected flow sensitivity is too high.

78 Filtering Images (to Reduce Artifacts)

A variety of filters are available for use on most MRI scanners to improve the appearance of images and minimize artifacts. Although the specific characteristics of each filter vary from vendor to vendor there are inherent similarities. Filters can be k-space based ("raw data filtering") or image based ("image data filtering"). Described below are several examples of filters designed to reduce artifacts associated with image acquisition and hardware limitations.

The first filter addresses artifacts associated with an incomplete digitization or truncation of the MR echo (see case 103). The artifact known as Gibbs' ringing or simply truncation artifact is visible as additional lines or ringing near the sharp changes in intensity at the edge of a volume of tissue or at an interface (e.g., air–skull, cord–CSF). Truncation artifacts arise from the failure to completely sample all spatial frequencies for an MR image. Thus this type of artifact is more conspicuous in lower resolution images (and more specifically along an axis with a large pixel dimension), and for that reason also often along the phase encoding direction. Filtering in k space for Gibbs' ringing is done using a bell-shaped filter such as a Hanning or Gaussian filter that essentially causes the echo to reach a zero signal point more rapidly and before the end of the acquisition window. The result is a dampening of the signal toward the edges of k space creating a smooth (nontruncated) transition.

The second example of a filter (for illustrations and further detail see case 97) deals with spatial distortion caused by imaging obtained at or near the edge of the usable field of view of the MRI hardware. This distortion can be caused by a change in the gradient linearity or falloff of the main B_0 field and can lead to a warping (distortion) of the ends of the image or signal loss at the edge of the field of view. The image-based filter applied in this instance (termed a "large field of view" filter by one manufacturer) attempts to correct for these changes, thus leading to a more accurate spatial representation of tissues—through calculations that measure the extent of and correct for spatial distortion. Although helpful, distortion correction filters do have limitations when the extent of distortion becomes severe. For example, spatial resolution is not maintained, and often poor, in areas of distortion. Users, therefore, should make every effort to position the body part being examined as close to the center of the main magnetic field as possible.

The third example of a filter is one that deals with variations in signal intensity across the field of view when multiple coil elements are used to obtain an image. This class of filters has assumed increased importance with the advent of multichannel phased array surface coils (see case 83). Variations in signal may be especially noticeable in the abdomen where tissues close to the coil elements in the anterior and posterior aspect of the body are bright but the center of the body far from the coil is dark due to insufficient coil element penetration. Signal normalization filters balance the pixel intensities between the bright pixels adjacent to the coil and darker pixels in the center of the image to create a more uniform intensity across the entire image. Fig. 78–1 depicts fat-suppressed fluid-attenuated inversion recovery (FLAIR) images acquired using an eight-channel coil without (Fig. 78–1A) and with (Fig. 78–1B)

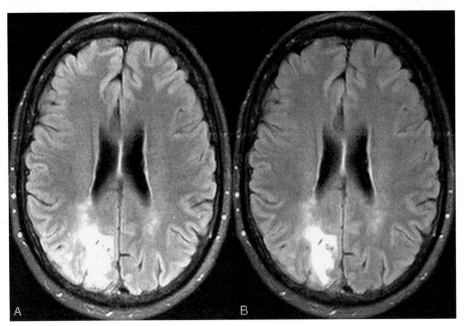

Figure 78–1

application of a normalization filter. Note the artificially increased signal intensity along the periphery of the brain in the unfiltered image, which makes windowing of the postoperative gliosis in the right occipital lobe difficult. The normalized image (Fig. **78–1B**) exhibits more uniform signal intensity across the field of view.

79 Filtering Images (to Improve SNR)

There are filters for MR that are designed to improve signal-to-noise ratio (SNR). As with all filters, there are two general types: k-space based and image based. Fig. **79–1A** illustrates the k-space data for a single slice acquisition, prior to application of a filter. Fig. **79–1B** shows the image following the application of an "elliptical" filter (so designated by one manufacturer), designed to reduce noise with minimal compromise in edge definition. The simple application of this or similar filters can increase SNR by 20%. Depending on vendor, the operator may or may not have control over the application of any filters, whether they be k-space or image based. If user selectable, k-space-based filters must be specified prior to image acquisition (as they are applied to the raw data).

Postprocessing (image-based) filters that reduce noise and improve the overall aesthetic appearance of images are applied after image acquisition and reconstruction, leading, if properly applied, to an improvement in SNR and overall image quality. Fig. **79–2** illustrates the application of a noise-reducing filter that assesses the randomness of conspicuous structures within the image to eliminate noise, thereby increasing SNR and improving the overall appearance of the image. The software takes into account the tissue structure continuity and signal intensity distribution to increase the accuracy in noise reduction.

Axial postcontrast T1-weighted images of the brain are illustrated in Fig. **79–2**. Fig. **79–2A–C** are from the same image acquisition, and differ only in postprocessing. No filter was applied in Fig. **79–2A**, a medium filter in Fig. **79–2B**, and a heavy filter in Fig. **79–2C**. Fig. **79–2D** shows an image from a separate scan, with twice the number of scan acquisitions and thus twice the scan time. Simply by processing the original image (Fig. **79–2A**) with a medium filter (Fig. **79–2B**), an improvement in SNR and

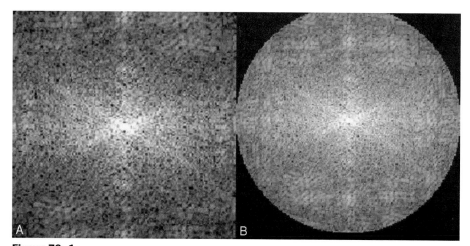

Figure 79–1

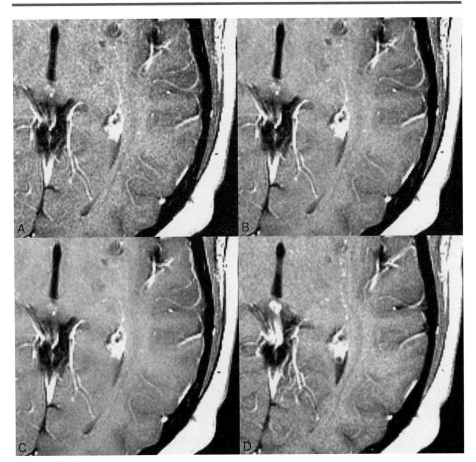

Figure 79–2

image quality is achieved similar to that possible by doubling the scan acquisitions (Fig. **79–2D**), but without the corresponding increase in acquisition time. Note the reduction in "graininess" of the image in Fig. **79–2B** as compared with Fig. **79–2A**. With a heavy filter (Fig. **79–2C**), there is a further reduction in noise, but also an artificial "smoothing" of the image. The use of postacquisition or postprocessing filters, as with all filters, varies by manufacturer—in type, degree, and transparency to the user. Some vendors allow the user to choose whether a filter is applied and its degree, whereas other vendors apply a standard filter without the knowledge of the user. Employed judiciously, postprocessing filters can improve overall image quality. It should be noted that increasing SNR by increasing the number of scan acquisitions has negatives other than simply scan time. The longer the scan, the greater is the chance for ghosting and blurring from inadvertent patient motion.

80 3D Evaluation: Image Postprocessing

Three-dimensional imaging techniques provide image data sets that can be further processed to create additional representations of the anatomy or pathology.

◆ Multiplanar Reconstruction (MPR)

With multiplanar reconstruction, images can be calculated for an infinite number of orientations within the acquired volume. The reconstruction is not necessarily restricted to planes, but can also be performed along curved cuts. Fig. **80–1** illustrates the midline sagittal image from a postcontrast 3D magnetization-prepared rapid gradient echo (MP-RAGE) acquisition (**A**), and a curved coronal reconstruction from the same data set (**B**).

◆ Maximum Intensity Projection (MIP)

In an MIP image, by definition, each pixel is assigned the highest observed signal from along the specified trajectory through the 3D data set. The user specifies the trajectory or perspective from which the 3D data set is thus viewed in 2D. Typically the data set is viewed from multiple angles, meaning that multiple MIPs are created for interpretation. A targeted MIP is one in which only part of the volume, typically containing the vessels of interest (when processing a 3D MRA data set), is used. The projection created from such a targeted volume contains less noise and fewer extraneous structures, significantly improving image quality.

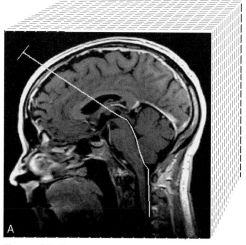
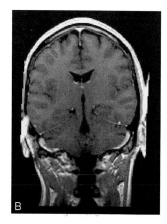

Figure 80–1

◆ Surface Shaded Display (SSD)

With surface shaded display, surfaces of volumes are reconstructed. A lower and an upper gray scale limit is defined by the user and the first value found along the trajectory from the user's view through the 3D image data set is declared the "surface." A virtual light source is used to modify the gray scale of the surface to create a 3D impression of the surface. Fig. **80–2A** presents the MIP and Fig. **80–2B** the SSD from a contrast-enhanced MRA exam, depicting a high-grade stenosis of the left subclavian artery with each respective postprocessing technique.

◆ Volume Rendering Technique (VRT)

Volume rendering involves choosing a particular signal intensity range or pixel values such that all other values can be considered as being transparent. The 3D effect is achieved by assigning a color to pixel values that match the defined range, using a color transition, transparency, or shading depending on position along the trajectory. In addition, a virtual light source can be used to outline the surfaces of the structures. The entire volume data set is included in the image. Areas of interest such as bone and blood vessels can be emphasized interactively by assigning appropriate color and transparency values. The VRT method is based on the idea that defined rendering properties (color, brightness, contrast, and transparency) are assigned to the voxels of the volume data set depending on the initial pixel value.

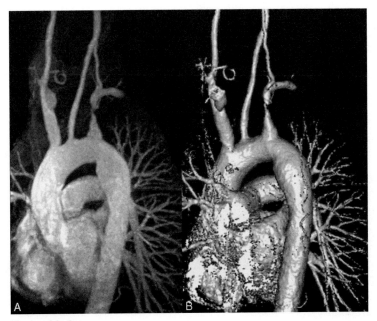

Figure 80–2

81 Parallel Imaging: k-Space-Based Reconstruction

Fig. **81–1** illustrates the underlying principles of a k-space-based parallel acquisition technique. Fourier transformation is able to differentiate between adjacent voxels if the transverse magnetization is pointing in opposite directions (*1* in Fig. **81–1**). That information is contained in the first Fourier line. To uniquely identify the origin of the signal, the next Fourier line is acquired with a lower phase encoding gradient amplitude, to acquire the change in phase for the transverse magnetization for a lower spatial resolution. If, to reduce measurement time, the measurement of every second Fourier line is omitted, the unique identification of the origin of the signal is no longer possible, leading to wraparound artifacts (see case 102) (*2* in Fig. **81–1**). The omission of the measurement of every second Fourier line corresponds to selecting a rectangular field of view or, as in this displayed case, deselecting the 100% oversampling in the direction of phase encoding.

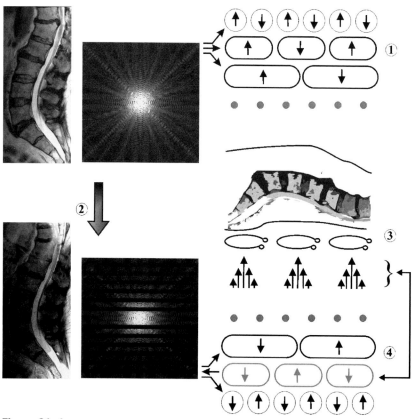

Figure 81–1

The spatial information of multiple surface coils distributed in the direction of phase encoding can be used to recover the information lost by omitting every second Fourier line. As illustrated by *3* in Fig. **81–1**, the signal intensity received by each coil shows an amplitude variation depending on the distance of the signal source from the coil. This amplitude variation contains the same spatial information that the phase modulation achieved with a phase-encoding gradient. Using combinations of the parallel-acquired coil signals, it is possible to employ this information to "reconstruct" the missing Fourier lines (*4* in Fig. **81–1**) and reestablish the uniqueness of signal assignment (eliminate wraparound artifacts). This is the underlying principle of k-space oriented parallel acquisition techniques like simultaneous acquisition of spatial harmonics (SMASH), parallel imaging with localized sensitivities (PILS), and generalized autocalibrating partially parallel acquisition (GRAPPA).

The fast spin echo T2-weighted sagittal scans of the lumbar spine in Fig. **81–2** were acquired without (Fig. **81–2A**) and with (Fig. **81–2B**) parallel imaging (the latter using GRAPPA). In Fig. **81–2B**, the measurement of every second Fourier line has been skipped [an integrated parallel acquisition technique (iPAT) factor of 2]. Scan time is thus reduced by a factor of two (comparing Fig. **81–2B** to Fig. **81–2A**). However, because each Fourier line contributes to the overall signal-to-noise ratio (SNR), there is a commensurate loss in SNR.

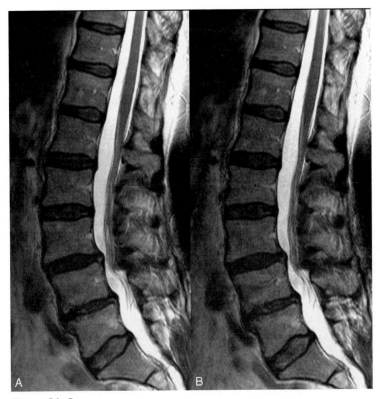

Figure 81–2

82 Parallel Imaging: Image-Based Reconstruction

The previous case illustrates the application of parallel imaging using k-space–based reconstruction. Parallel imaging can also be performed using image-based reconstruction. However, this approach has some disadvantages, as will be illustrated.

If there is a distribution of surface coils along the phase encoding direction, the separately reconstructed images, using the parallel acquired signals induced in each coil, will have wraparound artifacts (see case 102) that are position dependent (Fig. **82–1**). For example, in the image from coil 1 (*1* in Fig. **82–1**), the more caudal structures (pubic symphysis, bladder, sacrum) have substantial signal due to their proximity to the coil. This produces a prominent wraparound artifact in the image

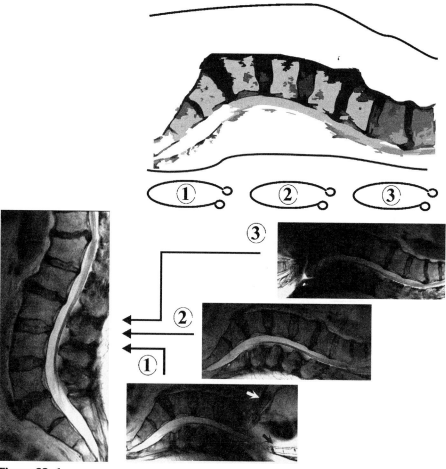

Figure 82–1

(*1* in Fig. **82–1**) overlying the upper lumbar spine (arrows). The same wraparound artifact is only faintly visible in the image from coil 2 (*2* in Fig. **82–1**) and nonexistent in the image from coil 3 (*3* in Fig. **82–1**).

Knowing the coil sensitivity, that is, the expected receiving range of each coil, the wraparound artifact can be mathematically identified and removed. This is the underlying principle of image-based parallel acquisition techniques like SENSE (SENSitivity Encoding).

Fig. **82–2** illustrates the application of SENSE. Fig. **82–2A** is a fast spin echo T2-weighted sagittal scan of the lumbar spine acquired without the use of parallel imaging. Fig. **82–2B** is using SENSE as the reconstruction algorithm, after omission of the measurement of every second Fourier line (parallel imaging with an iPAT factor of 2). Thus, the scan time for Fig. **82–2B** is half that of Fig. **82–2A**. SNR is also reduced, as anticipated, due to the reduction in number of phase encoding steps. However, note that there are residual wraparound artifacts (arrow, Fig. **82–2B**), a major drawback to the use of image-based reconstruction in parallel imaging.

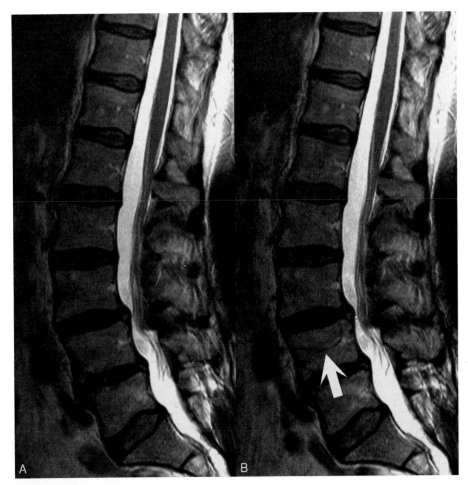

Figure 82–2

83 Parallel Imaging and Multichannel Coils

Speed of acquisition and signal-to-noise ratio (SNR) are closely related, critical parameters in the pursuit of diagnostic quality MR scans. Since MR's clinical introduction in the early 1980s, software and hardware advances have been consistently made, permitting faster and higher quality (improved spatial resolution and SNR) exams. A major early advance was the introduction of surface coils, which led eventually to the multichannel phased array systems available today. Surface coils offered improved SNR, but limited anatomic coverage, which was overcome by the use of carefully engineered combinations of surface coils. For example, attention has to be given to coil decoupling. Severe coupling between surface coils makes multiple coils operate as one large coil, and the benefits of a phased array is lost. The term *phased array* in reference to MR surface coils comes from radar and ultrasound, where a similar situation exists. To reduce the effects of coupling between coils, mutual inductance has to be minimized, for example, by using appropriate coil overlap, or alternatively by coil design with orthogonal modes (CP mode), and by isolation via separate preamplifiers. For an ideal orthogonal mode, effects of coupling are eliminated, noise correlation is zero, and there is no need for isolating preamplifiers. Thus different coil arrangements can be linked together creating different "modes."

The aim of all these arrangements is to maximize the SNR for the selected coil setup or to optimize regional coverage at some expense in SNR. One difficulty is that the detected signal is greater close to the coil as compared with areas further away. To deal with this problem, a normalization filter (see case 78) can be applied to the images to reduce the brightness of the areas in the near vicinity of the coil and increase the brightness in areas further away from the coil. Signal intensity appears more uniform across the image after application of such a normalization filter. However, the filter does not improve SNR, and more specifically in areas of low SNR further from the coil it is simply that the pixel signal intensity has been increased.

The variation in signal intensity due to each small coil element, however, can be used to identify the position of the coils, a prerequisite for parallel acquisition techniques. When employing parallel imaging, a prescan or a scan integrated into the measurement is acquired to provide the coil sensitivity profile. This profile is required to subsequently reconstruct the image, because knowledge of the coil profile is used to permit a reduction in the number of Fourier lines measured (the use of parallel imaging to reduce scan time, see case 7).

Fig. 83–1 depicts six images (around the periphery) that correspond to the images acquired from each coil element (using six elements in a multichannel phased array body coil), together with the single final reconstructed image in the center. On current clinical systems, only the final composite image is routinely provided for viewing, with the intermediate steps transparent to the user. A T1-weighted fat-suppressed spoiled gradient echo breath-hold technique was employed for image acquisition. Note the variation in signal intensity across each image from an individual coil element, with the signal (and SNR) highest close to the coil and falling off with increasing distance.

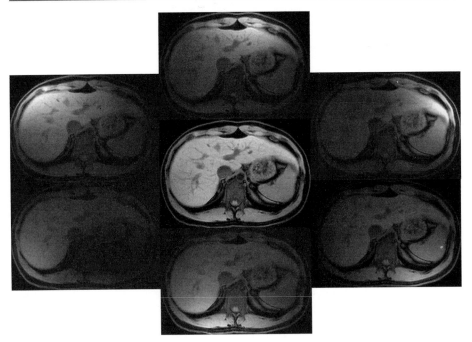

Figure 83–1

To take advantage of parallel imaging, coils need to be designed so that there are at least two elements in the direction of the intended imaging plane (and specifically the phase encoding direction). Clinical MR systems have recently been redesigned to make this possible for whole-body imaging, specifically allowing parallel acquisition in all three planes. It should also be kept in mind that although parallel imaging usually implies a reduction in SNR implicit with the decrease in scan time, this is not always the case. Parallel imaging when applied to echoplanar imaging (with a common clinical application being diffusion weighted scans) leads to reduced bulk susceptibility artifacts (and thus improved image quality) without a loss in SNR.

84 Contrast Media: Extracellular Agents (Gd Chelates)

The gadolinium chelates are the dominant class of contrast media for MRI. They are clear, colorless fluids, formulated without bacteriostatic additives for intravenous administration. The standard dose (excluding use in MR angiography) is 0.1 mmol/kg, which corresponds to 15 mL for a 75-kg patient (with all agents except one formulated at a concentration of 0.5 molar). The distribution of the agents is to the extracellular space.

Lesion enhancement occurs by one of two mechanisms: disruption of the blood–brain barrier (for intraaxial lesions) and lesion vascularity. The gadolinium ion is strongly paramagnetic, leading to a reduction in both T1 and T2, which is visualized on T1-weighted images as an increase in signal intensity. In Fig. **84–1**, thin section T1-weighted images are illustrated at the level of the internal auditory canal, revealing a soft tissue mass (an acoustic schwannoma) on the right precontrast (Fig. **84–1A**), which demonstrates prominent enhancement postcontrast (white arrow, Fig. **84–1B**). Enhancement of normal vascular structures includes the nasal turbinates (black arrow, Fig. **84–1B**) and choroid plexus, easily recognized markers of postcontrast scans. Clinically, contrast enhancement is used both for improved lesion detection and characterization. Major indications include neoplastic disease, infection, arteriovenous abnormalities, and, to a lesser degree, infarction. In recent years, the field of contrast-enhanced MR angiography has developed as an additional major application of the gadolinium chelates.

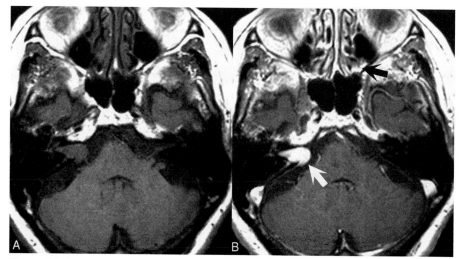

Figure 84–1

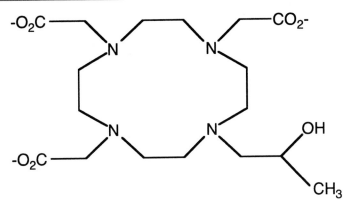

Figure 84–2

The word *chelate* comes from the Greek root *chelos*, meaning claw. The safety basis of the gadolinium chelates rests with the ability of the chelate to hold extremely tightly the gadolinium ion and assure near 100% excretion. Gadolinium is a heavy metal, a member of the transition elements (atomic number 64), and as such is extremely toxic in elemental form (Gd^{3+}). The gadolinium chelates are 100% renally excreted, with the exception of two agents with combined renal and hepatobiliary excretion [MultiHance and Gd ethoxybenzyl (EOB)–diethylenetriamine pentaacetic acid (DTPA)].

The gadolinium chelates currently available for clinical use can be differentiated on the basis of charge (ionic or nonionic), structure (linear or cyclic), and stability. Given that the gadolinium ion carries a +3 charge, if the ligand, for example, is that in Fig. **84–2** (HP-DO3A, the ligand for ProHance), the metal chelate itself will carry a net charge of zero, and thus be nonionic. In the U.S. market, considering only the gadolinium chelates with 100% renal excretion, there are one ionic agent (Magnevist) and three nonionic agents (ProHance, Omniscan, and Optimark). The structure of the chelate can be linear or cyclic (ring like, as seen in Fig. **84–2**), with the cyclic chelates demonstrating higher in vivo stability and thus theoretical safety margin. ProHance is the only cyclic chelate available in the U.S. Internationally, two other extracellular gadolinium chelates are in widespread use, both cyclic: Dotarem (ionic) and Gadovist (nonionic).

The gadolinium chelates, however, cannot be differentiated on the basis of major adverse reactions. All share a common safety profile, with nausea reported in 1.5% and urticaria in 0.5% of all injections. Health care personnel should be aware of the potential (although rare) for severe anaphylactoid reactions, with treatment identical to that for an iodinated contrast reaction. Patients with asthma, allergies, or known drug sensitivities (including allergy to iodinated contrast media) are at increased risk for a severe anaphylactoid reaction.

85 Contrast Media: Other Gadolinium Chelates

By slight changes in structure, agents with improved relaxivity and altered distribution have been developed. MultiHance, for example, has 40% higher relaxivity (equivalent to double dose) and partial hepatobiliary excretion, due to addition of a phenyl ($C_6H_5^-$) moiety. Fig. **85–1** illustrates the improved enhancement of a brain metastasis with MultiHance (Fig. **85–1B**) as compared with a conventional Gd^{3+} chelate (Fig. **85–1A**).

Fig. **85–2** illustrates a liver metastasis prior to (Fig. **85–2A**), immediately following (Fig. **85–2B**), and at 1 hour after (Fig. **85–2C**) MultiHance injection. Hepatobiliary

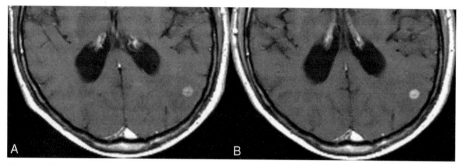

Figure 85–1

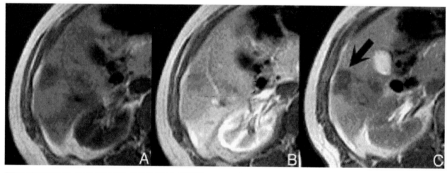

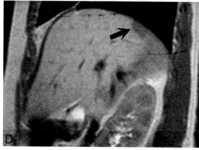

Figure 85–2

uptake and excretion of the agent are illustrated, with sustained enhancement of normal liver, opacification of the gallbladder, and slightly improved visualization of a liver metastasis (arrow) on the delayed image. High-quality breath-hold imaging in all three planes is possible in the hepatobiliary phase, providing improved detection of liver metastases, such as that seen immediately below the dome of the diaphragm (Fig. **85–2D**, arrow). Agents with very high hepatobiliary excretion [i.e., Gd ethoxybenzyl (EOB)–diethylenetriamine pentaacetic acid (DTPA), ~50%] and prolonged residence in the bloodstream (i.e., MS-325, mean half-life 16.3 hours), due to albumin binding, are currently subject to review by the respective health authorities in Europe and the United States.

Some of the newer gadolinium chelates have advantages as well in contrast-enhanced MR angiography. For example, vessel signal intensity has been shown to be 80% higher with MultiHance, as compared with more conventional agents. These improvements, together with technologic advances in equipment design, have made possible high-resolution whole-body 3D contrast-enhanced MR angiography (Fig. **85–3**, courtesy of Mathias Goyen, MD), with five 3D data sets, slightly overlapping, acquired in immediate succession following a single intravenous contrast dose. Fig. **85–4** illustrates patient positioning and image acquisition for three such image sets.

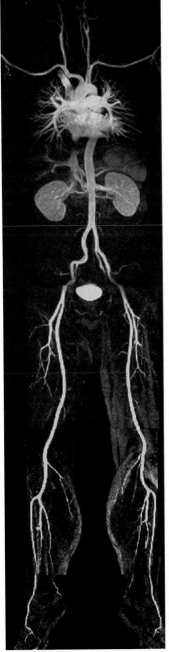

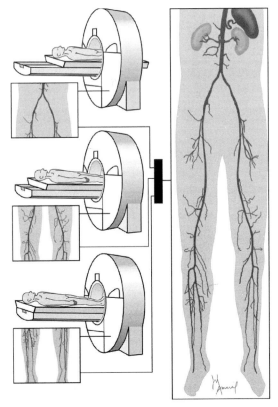

Figure 85–3   **Figure 85–4**

86 Contrast Media: Other Agents (Non-Gadolinium)

Other contrast media, not based on gadolinium, have also been developed for MRI. Superparamagnetic iron particles are selectively taken up following intravenous injection by Kupffer cells, primarily in the liver. Two such iron oxide–based agents are approved: ferumoxides (Endorem, distributed in the United States as Feridex), with a particle size range of 50 to 180 nm, and Resovist (not available in the U.S.), with a particle size of ~60 nm. The principal relaxation effect of these larger particles is on T2 (due to susceptibility effects, with the contrast agent causing a decrease in signal intensity), with scans performed in a delayed fashion postinjection, allowing time for liver uptake. Resovist is also approved for bolus injection (dynamic imaging), with T1-weighted scans and positive contrast enhancement noted in this application. The safety profile for Feridex is not comparable to that of the gadolinium chelates, with a substantially higher incidence of adverse reactions. Resovist is more recently approved and has an improved safety profile.

In Fig. **86–1**, imaging with Resovist reveals a hypervascular lesion on Fig. **86–1A**, the dynamic scan, with prominent iron uptake on Fig. **86–1B**, the delayed scan (white arrow), compatible with an adenoma. In Fig. **86–2**, the precontrast in-phase T1-weighted scan (Fig. **86–2A**) reveals a cirrhotic, nodular liver. On Fig. **86–2B**, the delayed postcontrast scan (using Resovist), a subcapsular hepatocellular carcinoma (white arrow) and multiple low signal intensity regenerating liver nodules (black arrows) can be identified (images courtesy of Drs. Schoenberg, Michaely, and Zech, University of Munich–Grosshadern Hospitals, Germany).

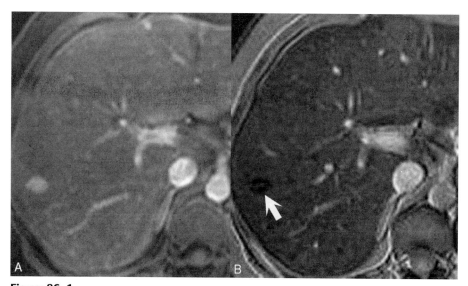

Figure 86–1

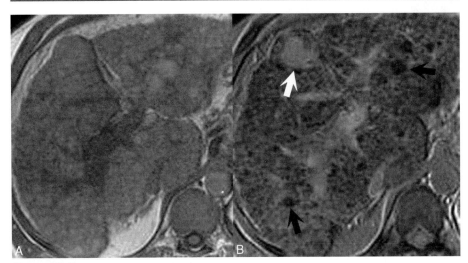

Figure 86–2

Teslascan, a manganese (Mn) based agent, was approved in the late 1990s. Unlike the gadolinium chelates, this agent dissociates after IV injection, yielding free Mn. Safety concerns persist due to this release. Like Feridex, the incidence of adverse events is substantially higher as compared with the Gd chelates. T1-weighted images are employed postcontrast (with Mn having paramagnetic properties similar to Gd, but of lower magnitude), with approval limited to delayed liver imaging.

Oral MR contrast agents are classified according to the observed signal intensity (SI): positive ("bright" lumen), negative ("dark" lumen), or biphasic. Several agents are commercially available in various (but not all) countries, with utilization in general low. Positive agents originally included dilutions of the gadolinium chelates, specifically formulated for oral use (these are no longer available commercially), and solutions of iron or manganese ions. Some natural substances, such as milk, vegetable oil, green tea, and blueberry juice, and some manufactured products, such as ice cream, also act as positive oral contrast agents, due to either high fat or manganese ion content. Agents containing manganese typically are biphasic in character, with high SI on T1- and low SI on T2-weighted images. Negative contrast agents, which provide a dark lumen on both T1- and T2-weighted images, include several different iron particulate preparations (for example, Lumirem). Water can be used as an oral contrast agent, but its use is limited by intestinal resorption. Barium sulfate can also provide some luminal contrast, with SI (low on T1 and low to high on T2) dependent on administered concentration and subsequent dilution.

87 Cardiac Imaging: Morphology

The application of MRI techniques to image rapidly moving objects such as the heart requires that conventional imaging methods be adapted to "freeze" normal cardiac motion while maintaining high spatial resolution. Rapid scan techniques such as HASTE (Fig. **87–1A**) (see case 22) and trueFISP (Fig. **87–1B**) (see case 30) provide excellent motion suppression with good spatial resolution. However, these rapid acquisition methods do not always provide the optimal T1 or T2 contrast required for the diagnosis of cardiac pathology.

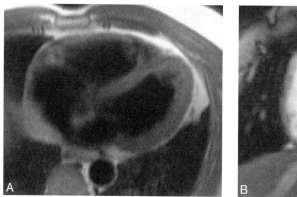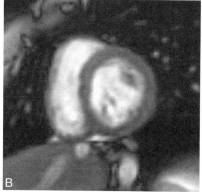

Figure 87–1

Routine spin echo (SE) and fast spin echo (FSE) images of a moving object such as the heart acquired in the standard fashion would demonstrate motion artifacts due to the rapid changes in the spatial location of cardiac tissues during the normal cardiac cycle. However, because the normal cardiac cycle is consistent and contains periods of little to no motion, termed diastole, standard sequences can be modified to acquire information only during these times. This process is called cardiac triggering and involves acquiring one echo associated with one line of k space (SE) or one echo train length (FSE) per diastolic period until all of k space is filled for one slice, resulting in good T1 or T2 contrast and high spatial resolution.

In certain instances, the bright signal from blood can obscure anatomic structures and hinder diagnosis. To remove the blood signal on morphologic images of the

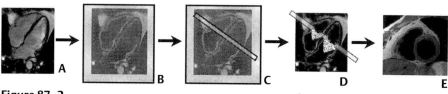

Figure 87–2

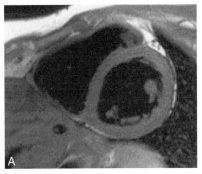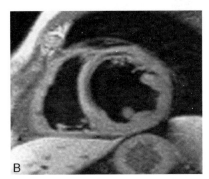

Figure 87-3

heart a process called double inversion recovery (IR) is employed. This process, depicted in Fig. **87-2**, involves the application of two inversion radiofrequency (RF)
pulses, prior to the standard RF pulses, to form an echo and results in images with the
signal from blood suppressed. The first IR pulse is nonselective and inverts all the hydrogen nuclei within the imaging field (Fig. **87-2B**). The second IR pulse is selective
and reinverts only those hydrogen nuclei within the selected slice plane, making a
normal slice acquisition possible (Fig. **87-2C**). The reinverted blood quickly flows out
of the slice plane and is replaced by inverted blood that has not been subjected to all
of the RF pulses (Fig. **87-2D**) and therefore does not contribute to the final image, resulting in an image without the signal contribution from blood (Fig. **87-2E**).

Fig. **87-3** depicts T1, segmented fast spin echo acquisitions of the heart in the
short axis orientation with double IR preparation pulses used for suppression of the
blood signal. Fig. **87-3B** incorporates, in addition, spectral fat suppression.

Fig. **87-4** presents segmented, FSE acquisitions incorporating double IR depicting
the left ventricular outflow tract (Fig. **87-4A**) and the thoracic aorta in its entirety
(Fig. **87-4B**) (using an oblique acquisition plane).

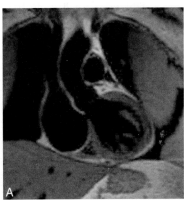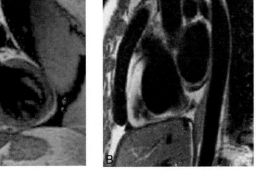

Figure 87-4

88 Cardiac Imaging: Function

Case 87 demonstrated that MRI is capable of showing structural (morphologic) information concerning the heart, with good tissue contrast and spatial resolution, while suppressing blood signal and artifacts associated with motion. However, a more complete analysis of the heart with MRI requires that information regarding the efficiency of cardiac function be obtained as well. Functional MRI of the heart requires another set of specially adapted sequences and postprocessing software.

In morphologic imaging a certain number of echoes associated with lines of k space are acquired during the diastolic phase of several cardiac cycles until a complete image is obtained. Functional sequences work much in the same way. In functional cardiac imaging, the complete cardiac cycle is divided into a specific number of phases. During each phase a certain number of echoes associated with lines of k space are generated and the process is performed over the number of cardiac cycles necessary to complete an image of each phase of the cycle. The images are viewed in a cine loop resulting in a visual representation of the complete cardiac cycle for that slice position (Fig. **88–1A**).

Additional information, including specifically cardiac output and ejection fraction, can be extracted from these functional images with simple volume analysis

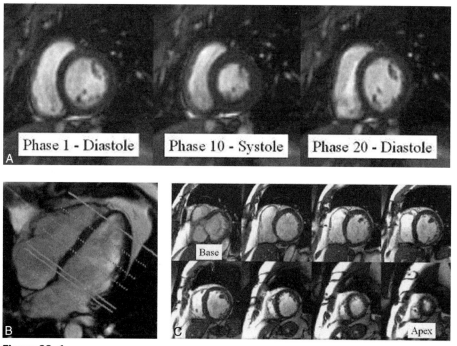

Figure 88–1

software. To accomplish this task, functional slices of the entire cardiac cycle are acquired contiguously to cover the complete volume of the right or left ventricle (Fig. **88–1B,C**).

The volume of blood within the slice during each phase is calculated (Fig. **88–2A**), and the volume from each slice across the ventricle added together, resulting in a quantitative analysis of the volume of blood within the entire ventricle during systole and diastole. Fig. **88–2B** depicts the slice volumes from the end diastolic phase (ED) and the end systolic phase (ES) that are added together to calculate the volume of the entire ventricle (Fig. **88–2C**). This information is then used to calculate specific indicators of cardiac efficiency (Fig. **88–2D**).

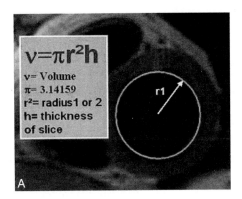

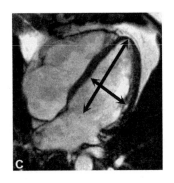

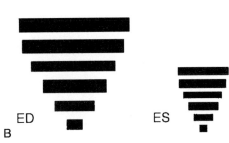

ED

ES

B

C

Stroke Volume = EDV – ESV

Cardiac Output = SV x HR / 1000

EF = ((EDV – ESV) / EDV) x 100

Where:
EDV = End Diastolic Volume
ESV = End Systolic Volume
SV = Stroke Volume
HR = Heart Rate
EF = Ejection Fraction   D

Figure 88–2

89 Cardiac Imaging: Myocardial Perfusion

Occlusions or constrictions within the arteries supplying blood to the cardiac muscle can lead to a reduction in or cessation of the flow of oxygenated blood reaching the myocardium, thereby inhibiting the supply of nutrients necessary for cellular activity and normal cardiac function. The MR approach used to assess the extent and uniformity of microvascular blood flow to the myocardium is referred to as cardiac perfusion imaging. Multislice, T1-weighted scans are acquired through the left ventricle within each cardiac cycle before, during, and after bolus administration of a contrast agent that decreases T1, such as a gadolinium chelate. The process provides a dynamic assessment of the rate and extent of blood with a short T1 perfusing the left ventricle and can be analyzed both visually and with postprocessing software.

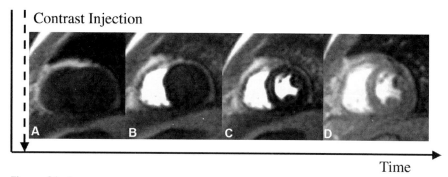

Figure 89–1

Fig. **89–1** demonstrates four time points of a perfusion data set acquired in the short-axis orientation through the middle of the left ventricle. The first image (Fig. **89–1A**) shows very little structural information as the bolus of contrast agent has yet to arrive within the slice. Fig. **89–1B** and **C** depict a dramatic signal increase, representing the arrival of contrast within the right ventricle, and then slightly later in time also within the left ventricle. However, the left ventricular muscle itself has yet to receive the T1-shortened blood and therefore remains dark. Fig. **89–1D** shows the signal increase within the left ventricular myocardium, which corresponds to perfusion of the muscle by blood containing the gadolinium chelate. The entire data set is observed and analyzed for areas showing a decrease in the rate or an absence of signal change during the perfusion study.

Several postprocessing techniques are available, and methods vary from vendor to vendor. The following example represents a simple mean intensity perfusion analysis. Fig. **89–2A** depicts one time point in a perfusion data set where three regions of interest (ROIs) have been drawn. The ROIs are propagated to the entire set of

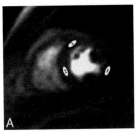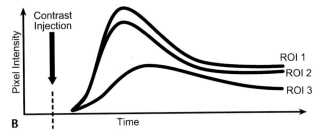

Figure 89–2

time points from this slice position, and the changes in pixel intensity for each region are mapped over time as demonstrated in Fig. **89–2B**.

Rapidly acquired, gradient echo sequences are used to allow for a full, multislice acquisition in every heartbeat. Spatial resolution is adjusted based on each patient's specific heart rate. The procedure is often duplicated before and after the administration of myocardial stress agents that increase the contraction force of the heart, giving a more thorough assessment of the extent of cardiac perfusion.

Fig. **89–3A** demonstrates early perfusion of the left ventricle as viewed in the four-chamber or horizontal long axis orientation. Fig. **89–3B** depicts perfusion viewed in the short axis orientation, demonstrating, in a different patient, a delay in the perfusion of the inferior (or "posterior") wall of the left ventricle at the midventricular level (arrows).

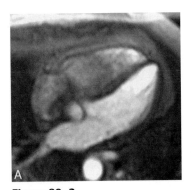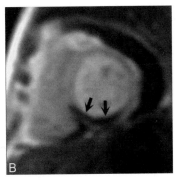

Figure 89–3

90 Cardiac Imaging: Myocardial Viability

Myocardial muscle tissue that has been damaged by a reduction in the normal flow of oxygenated blood falls into three main categories. The first category, stunned myocardium, is living, viable tissue that has been subjected to short durations of reduced blood flow. In most cases, stunned myocardium will recover to normal function with time. The second category, hibernating myocardium, is that which has been subjected to long durations of reduced blood flow and requires interventional measures to restore normal cardiac function. The third category is necrotic or nonviable myocardium, tissue that no longer contains living myocardial cells or myocytes and therefore is unable to be returned to normal function. Patients with known cardiomyopathy resulting from decreased blood flow to the myocardium may benefit greatly from interventional measures if the area in question remains viable. However, if the tissue is no longer viable, there is little benefit in subjecting the patient to the possible risks of an interventional procedure. The differentiation between viable and nonviable myocardium is the focus of cardiac viability MRI.

The gadolinium chelates are distributed following intravenous injection to the extracellular space, and thus to normal myocardium. Likewise, their concentration rapidly diminishes, after an early peak following injection, due to renal excretion and redistribution. However, in nonviable myocardial tissue, there is impaired washout of the contrast agent. Myocardial tissue that is nonviable becomes hyperintense on delayed T1-weighted scans after contrast injection, due to accumulation of gadolinium chelate. Hyperenhancement is seen in both acute and chronic infarction, but not in reversible ischemic injury, with histology revealing the enhancing areas to represent myocyte necrosis and collagenous scar.

The imaging approach involves the use of T1-weighted, gradient echo sequences incorporating an inversion pulse set to the inversion time (TI) necessary to suppress normal myocardial tissue. After administration of the contrast agent, the inversion time is decreased (relative to the value used precontrast) to properly suppress normal myocardial muscle, which now has a shorter T1 due to the presence of the contrast agent. The TI is adjusted throughout the exam based on the amount of time that has passed since contrast administration to maintain the level of myocardial suppression. Imaging begins approximately 5 to 20 minutes after the administration of contrast, to allow sufficient time for the agent to begin to accumulate within nonviable myocardium. The result is a substantial difference in tissue signal intensity between the suppressed normal myocardial muscle and enhanced areas of necrosis or scar.

Fig. **90–1** illustrates viability scan sequences acquired after intravenous contrast administration. Fig. **90–1A** demonstrates endocardial hyperenhancement (arrows) within the lateral wall of the left ventricle on a horizontal long axis slice. Fig. **90–1B** depicts another positive viability study with hyperenhancement of the apex and superior and inferior walls of the left ventricle displayed on a vertical long axis image. Fig. **90–1C** displays the results of a septal infarct, with corresponding myocardial muscle hyperenhancement. Fig. **90–1D** demonstrates hyperenhancement within the apex on a three-chamber view with associated thinning of the myocardium.

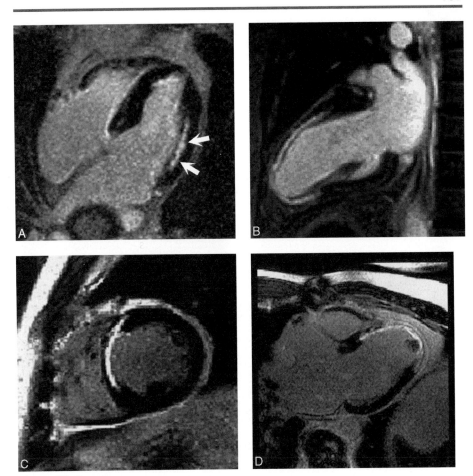

Figure 90–1

91 MR Mammography: Dynamic Imaging

In MRI of the breast, there is significant overlap in T1 and T2 between benign and malignant lesions, with these parameters thus of little utility. The introduction of dynamic postcontrast imaging represented a major breakthrough for diagnosis of breast tumors. This approach, however, requires advanced hardware and software. A dedicated double breast coil is mandatory, with newer designs also permitting MR-guided stereotactic biopsy. Both breasts need to be covered in a dynamic fashion with a slice thickness of ≈2 mm and in plane resolution ≤ 1 mm, placing considerable demands upon pulse sequence design. 3D gradient echo sequences are employed with a

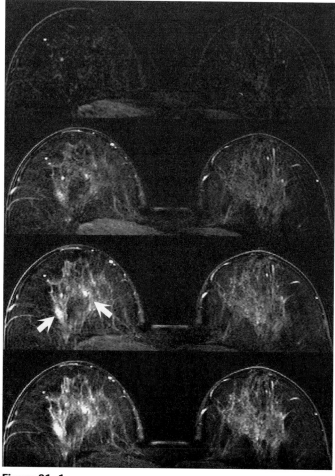

Figure 91–1

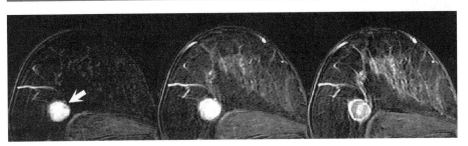

Figure 91–2

temporal resolution of ≈1 minute, imaging for ≈5 minutes following intravenous gadolinium chelate administration. To eliminate the high signal intensity of fat, subtraction of the unenhanced images from the contrast-enhanced images is performed (as in the scans illustrated). Alternatively, fat saturation or selective water excitation may be employed. Premenopausal women should be imaged between days 6 and 16 of the menstrual cycle. Otherwise enhancement of normal tissue due to hormonal stimulation may obscure or mimic malignant lesions. MR findings indicative of malignancy include irregular lesion contour, enhancement that follows ducts or starts from the periphery, and early lesion enhancement followed by a plateau or washout. In Fig. **91–1**, four dynamic scans are displayed (immediate, and 1, 3, and 5 minutes postcontrast). In the right breast (arrows), there are areas with prominent, fast enhancement, demonstrating some plateau, and thus suspicious for malignancy (invasive ductal carcinoma by surgical pathology). In Fig. **91–2**, three dynamic scans (immediate, and 1 and 3 minutes postcontrast) through a large malignant lymph node (arrow) in the same patient depict several typical signs of malignancy—a focal lesion with fast, prominent enhancement and early washout. Region-of-interest (quantitative) analysis is typically performed to evaluate the time course of enhancement, as illustrated in Fig. **91–3**. Due to overlap in contrast-enhancement patterns between benign and malignant lesions, interpretation of MR scans must be performed with correlation to x-ray mammography.

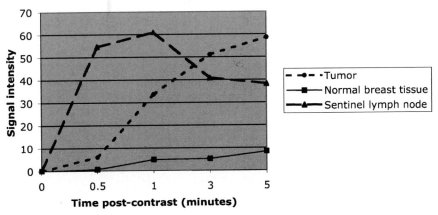

Figure 91–3

92   MR Mammography: Silicone

Fig. **92–1** presents multiple axial images from a silicone breast implant MR exam, together with a single sagittal image through the left breast. The imaging sequence employed both water and fat suppression, with silicone depicted as high signal intensity. Both implants demonstrate infolding of the silicone envelope, with silicone outside the envelope but contained within the fibrous capsule (a bilateral encapsulated leak,

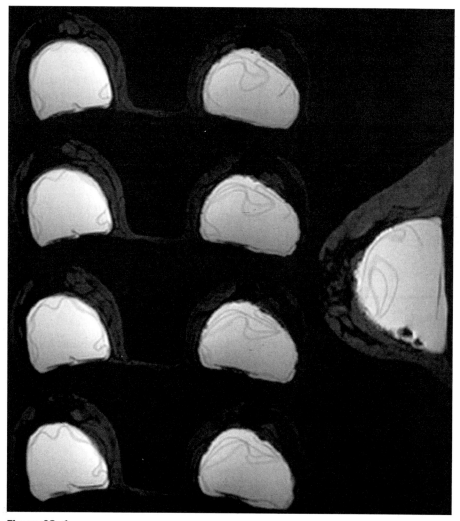

Figure 92–1

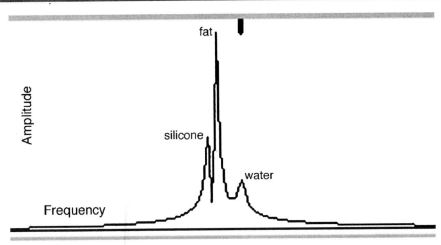

Figure 92–2

also known as an intracapsular rupture). The most reliable indicator of implant rupture on MR is the wavy line or "linguine" sign. Well seen in the left breast, this sign is characterized by multiple thin curvilinear lines within the implant, corresponding to the collapsed implant shell surrounded by silicone.

The main indication for MR of breast implants is for evaluation of possible rupture involving a silicone gel-filled implant. If rupture of an implant is detected, the amount and location of silicone within the soft tissues should be reported.

In the imaging of implants, 2D inversion recovery sequences (using fast spin echo technique, see case 17) are typically employed. The inversion time, TI, can be set for either fat suppression (TI ≈ 100 ms at 1.5 T) or for silicone suppression (TI ≈ 400 ms at 1.5 T). To depict silicone only (as in Fig. **92–1**), the signal from both fat and water must be suppressed. This is accomplished by employing an inversion recovery sequence (with TI set for fat suppression, see case 54) in combination with a spectral water suppression pulse (like that employed for spectral fat saturation, see case 52, but with the radiofrequency (RF) pulse applied prior to the spin preparation excitation set at the specific resonant frequency of water, thus saturating the spins at this frequency). Excellent homogeneity of the main magnetic field is a prerequisite for this approach. To achieve water suppression, the technologist adjusts the MR frequency of the scanner to the resonance frequency of water. In a plot of amplitude versus frequency (Fig. **92–2**), when displaying the MR spectra, three peaks will be seen (from left to right silicone, fat, and water). The fat peak is ≈3.3 ppm lower and the silicone peak (which normally slightly overlaps the fat peak) ≈4.5 ppm lower than the water peak. The pulse sequence, with spectral saturation thus set to the resonance frequency of water, is then initiated.

93 Artifacts: Magnetic Susceptibility

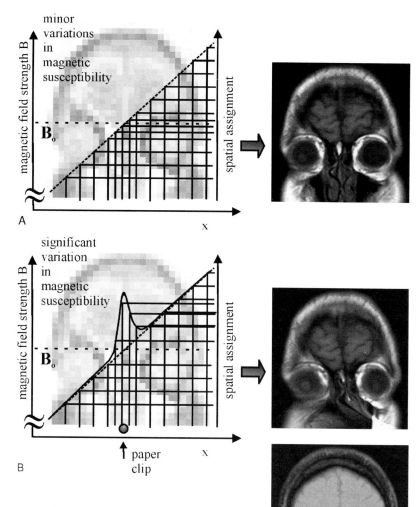

Figure 93–1

All matter is made up out of atoms, with each atom composed in part of electrons in motion. The currents associated with this motion generate a magnetization within the tissue. The relation of this magnetization with an external magnetic field is given by the magnetic susceptibility. If the magnetic susceptibility of the material is negative, the matter is called diamagnetic and the magnetic field in the presence of the material is weakened. If the magnetic susceptibility of the matter is positive, the material is called paramagnetic and the magnetic field is strengthened by the presence of the material. Ferromagnetic materials show a nonlinear dependence between magnetization and external field with a possible permanent magnetization and a significant amplification of the external field. The difference in magnetic susceptibility between different tissues is called a susceptibility gradient and may cause local magnetic field inhomogeneities, resulting in a nonlinear distribution of resonance frequencies. As magnetic field gradients are used for spatial encoding, any nonlinear distribution causes image distortion and artificial signal variations. Fig. **93–1** presents the consequences of a significant jump in magnetic susceptibility. Fig. **93–1A** shows the normal image appearance with minor variations in magnetic susceptibility within the tissue and a linear relationship between location and local magnetic field gradient. Fig. **93–1B** shows the effect of a paper clip placed between the teeth. The magnetic dipole formed by the ferromagnetic material changes the magnetic field far beyond the paper clip itself. Said in a different way, the field is strengthened far beyond and around the ferromagnetic object. The image reconstruction assumes a linear relationship between magnetic field and location, leading to displaced anatomy according to the strengthened (higher) magnetic field. Because less tissue is available with the expected resonance frequency in the immediate vicinity of the paper clip, the signal for this region is significantly reduced. Further away from the ferromagnetic object, this effect vanishes and finally the signal of the tissue within the area of a strengthened magnetic field constructively interferes with signal from tissue with the same resonance frequency, resulting in a hyperintense appearance at that location.

The nonlinearity of the magnetic field gradient caused by any ferromagnetic material has consequences beyond its effect on frequency encoding. The field gradient responsible for the slice selection is influenced as well, causing a significantly distorted slice profile. Furthermore, in gradient echo imaging the substantial differences in resonance frequencies confined to a very small location causes rapid phase dispersion leading to a large signal void (Fig. **93–1C**).

The sensitivity of gradient echo sequences for demonstrating the presence of susceptibility gradients (for example with hemorrhagic lesions) can be further enhanced by allowing more time for the dephasing process (using a longer echo time). This can be combined with an approach to increase the signal-to-noise ratio (SNR), because a low bandwidth sequence (which has higher SNR) requires a prolonged acquisition window, which results in a prolonged echo time.

Fig. **93–2** illustrates the effect of changing the bandwidth using pulse sequence diagrams. For a given slice selection gradient (GS), RF pulse, and phase encoding gradient (GP), lowering the bandwidth leads to an increase in the acquisition window and a longer TE. The frequency range across the field of view (FOV) in the readout direction is termed the sequence or image bandwidth. The span of frequencies across a single pixel is also commonly referred to as the bandwidth, which can be confusing, but is given in Hz/pixel. The noise in an image is distributed evenly across all frequencies. It thus follows that if the frequency range of the measurement is smaller (as with low bandwidth imaging), the noise is less (and thus the SNR higher).

Compartmentalization of paramagnetic deoxy- or methemoglobin inside intact red blood cells adjacent to nonparamagnetic plasma, as well as the presence of hemosiderin within soft tissues, gives rise to a susceptibility gradient resulting in significant $T2^*$ shortening. The sensitivity of a sequence to magnetic susceptibility effects increases with echo time. A low bandwidth sequence intrinsically has a longer TE and therefore is more sensitive to susceptibility gradients as well as providing higher SNR.

This is illustrated in Fig. **93–3**, with high (Fig. **93–3A**) and low (Fig. **93–3B**) bandwidth gradient echo images. There are large bilateral subacute subdural hematomas. The presence of hemoglobin breakdown products, and the susceptibility effect therein, is

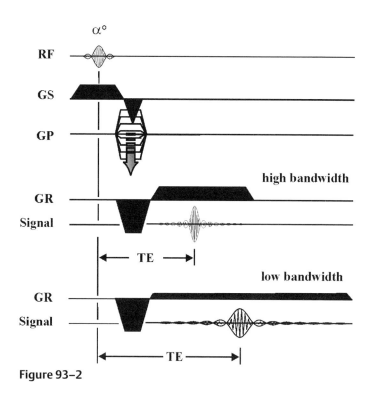

Figure 93–2

well demonstrated due to the associated low signal intensity (within the subdural collections bilaterally) on the low bandwidth image. This finding is not evident on the high bandwidth image. The SNR is also higher for the low bandwidth image.

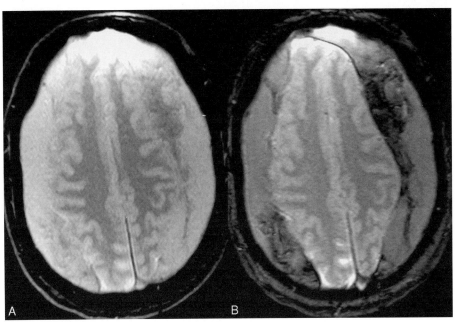

Figure 93–3

94 Maximizing Magnetic Susceptibility

Fig. **94–1** presents images of a cavernous angioma using several different scan techniques. On the SE sagittal T1-weighted image (Fig. **94–1A**), there is a mixture of signal intensities (arrow) due to coexistence of different stages of hemoglobin oxidation. The fast spin echo (FSE) T2-weighted (Fig. **94–1B**) and fluid-attenuated inversion recovery (FLAIR) (Fig. **94–1C**) scans exhibit signal loss due to hemosiderin in the left frontal white matter. The signal loss is much more prominent on the 2D gradient echo (GRE) scan (Fig. **94–1D**, arrow). T2* contrast is markedly improved in GRE scans

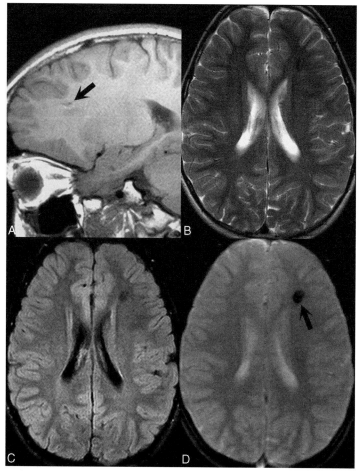

Figure 94–1

due to phase dispersion from local gradient effects. This results in a clearly demarcated area of signal loss, increasing the sensitivity for detection of such lesions.

The appearance of hemorrhage varies in a temporal fashion from the hyperacute stage (less than 24 hours) to the chronic stage (greater than 14 days). Visualization of hemorrhage varies even further depending on the anatomic compartment within which it occurs. Within a parenchymal hemorrhage, blood takes several different forms, with the temporal progression being that from oxyhemoglobin to deoxyhemoglobin, intracellular methemoglobin, extracellular methemoglobin, and eventually hemosiderin. Hemorrhage on T1-weighted scans in the hyperacute and acute stages is isointense to hypointense due to the long T1 imposed by a relatively high water content. As deoxyhemoglobin is transformed into methemoglobin, T1 is shortened (leading to high signal intensity) due to water's ability to interact with the paramagnetic ferric iron within methemoglobin.

Visualization of hemorrhage on T2-weighted scans is less straightforward. In a region of hemorrhage, the presence of paramagnetic blood breakdown products cause areas of varying magnetic susceptibilities and thus magnetic nonuniformity. Magnetic susceptibility is a measure of the ability of an object or substance to become magnetized in a magnetic field. In mathematical terms, it is defined as the ratio of induced magnetic field to applied magnetic field. Due to variability in magnetic susceptibility, there are static local field gradients that cause loss of phase coherence. Along with clot retraction, these phenomena effectively reduce T2 to a value known as $T2^*$ (T2 star), causing signal loss in regions of acute (deoxyhemoglobin), early subacute (intracellular methemoglobin), and chronic hemorrhage (hemosiderin and ferritin).

As with the visualization of metal artifacts (see case 95), the extent of signal loss is dependent on the selection of scan technique and imaging parameters. In imaging hemorrhage, however, it is at times useful to increase signal loss ($T2^*$ contrast) to improve lesion detection. FSE exams correct for phase dispersion due to local field gradients because of the use of a 180° RF pulse. In distinction, gradient echo scans do not correct for such phase dispersion. This results in increased signal loss and therefore increased sensitivity to detecting hemorrhage (better $T2^*$ contrast). $T2^*$ contrast may also be exaggerated by the use of a long TE, larger voxel size, and higher field strengths. With optimization of $T2^*$ contrast, 2D GRE scans may reveal hemorrhages not seen on fast spin echo. However, signal loss from $T2^*$ effects may also obscure adjacent brain structures, may be mistaken for other pathology, and may even make characterization of the hemorrhage itself difficult. In clinical practice, therefore, fast spin echo and 2D gradient echo scans complement one another in the visualization of hemorrhage.

95 Artifacts: Metal

The images presented show the artifact from a nonferromagnetic aneurysm clip. Spin echo (Fig. **95–1A**) and fast spin echo (Fig. **95–1B**) sequences have less distortion due to the presence of a 180° refocusing pulse, in comparison to gradient echo (GRE) sequences (Fig. **95–1D**). Fig. **95–1C** is a diffusion-weighted image (DWI) (see case 59), which of all techniques should show the greatest distortion. However, in this instance, parallel imaging has been employed with the result being substantially reduced artifact. The source image (Fig. **95–1E**) for the 3D time of flight (TOF) (see case 42) circle of Willis scan [maximum intensity projection (MIP), Fig. **95–1F**] utilizes a short TE and small voxels that decrease the area of the artifact when compared with the 2D GRE scan (Fig. **95–1D**). Note that the left anterior cerebral artery, left middle cerebral artery, and left proximal posterior cerebral artery are not seen (Fig. **95–1F**). Without viewing the source image (Fig. **95–1E**), one may not realize that nonvisualization of these vessels is due to artifact.

Ferromagnetic and nonferromagnetic materials can cause significant artifacts in MRI. The severity of the artifact correlates with the degree of ferromagnetism. Metal artifact may appear on MR in three ways: geometrical image distortion, especially at the boundaries of the object; gradual or distinct signal void around the object; and areas of sharply defined high signal intensity adjacent to the object.

Ferromagnetic materials directly distort the overall magnetic field in the area of the metal. Thus, the unique resonant frequency created by the gradients to encode spatial data is adversely changed. This results in spatial misrepresentation and therefore artifact. Nonferromagnetic materials, on the other hand, cause image distortion in two ways. The difference in magnetic susceptibility (see case 93) between the metal and the surrounding tissue causes a local magnetic field gradient. In addition, turning on and off gradient magnetic fields causes currents to flow in the metallic object (eddy currents) that further change the local magnetic field. These combined effects on the magnetic field create artifact via the same mechanism as with ferromagnetic objects.

Metal artifact can be accentuated or diminished depending on the imaging sequence and scan technique. Smaller voxels (see case 11), although unable to change the actual spatial extent of artifact, generally decrease the representation of artifact on the image seen by the radiologist. In addition, a long TE (echo time) and low sampling bandwidth provide a longer period of time for the metal to effect the image. A long interecho interval also increases the likelihood for spatial distortion to occur. Thus, choosing a scan with small voxels, a short TE, a short interecho interval, or a high sampling bandwidth decreases the severity of the artifact seen on the image.

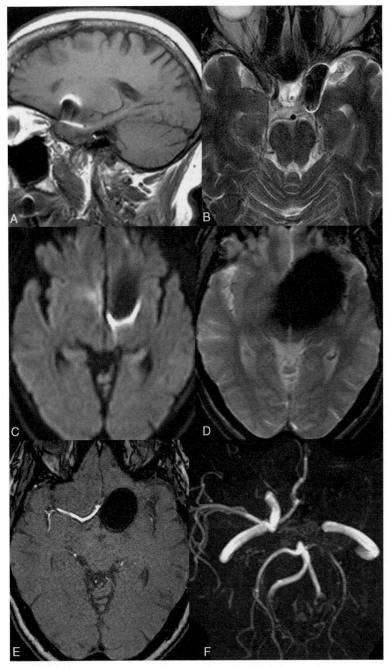

Figure 95–1

96 Chemical Shift Artifact: Sampling Bandwidth

Chemical shift, a common artifact, is seen in the readout direction. This artifact occurs at tissue interfaces with significantly different fat and water contents. In Fig. **96–1** and **96–2** the readout direction was top to bottom. The bandwidth of a pulse sequence (given in hertz/pixel on each image), specified prior to scan acquisition, controls the magnitude of the effect. The lower the bandwidth, the more prominent the artifact. Chemical shift appears on images as the presence of artifactual bright (black arrows) or dark (white arrows) lines at the fat/water interface (Fig. **96–1**) or by displacement of the water image relative to the fat image (Fig. **96–2**). In Fig. **96–2B**, the brain appears displaced posteriorly relative to the fat of the scalp and diploic space,

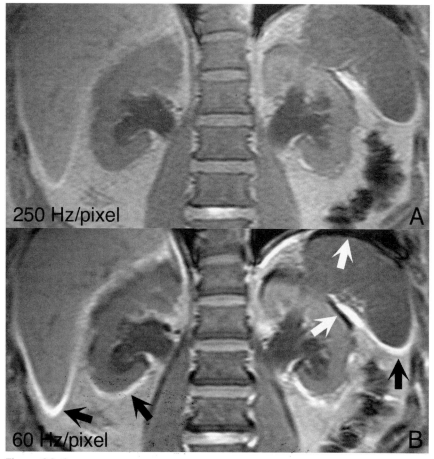

Figure 96–1

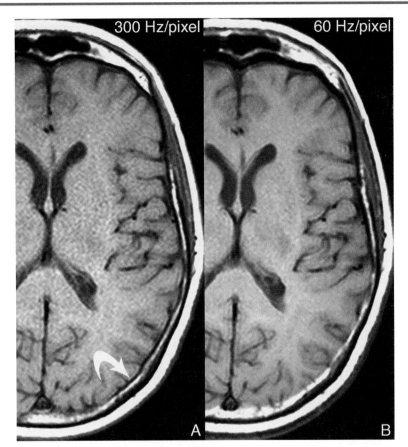

Figure 96–2

with the inner table of the skull (curved arrow, Fig. **96–2A**) no longer visible posteriorly on the low bandwidth image (Fig. **96–2B**). Depending on MR vendor, bandwidth may be specified in Hz/pixel, or by the total frequency range that is uniquely encoded (the Nyquist bandwidth). For example, when an image is acquired with a 130 Hz/pixel bandwidth, a 256 image has a full image bandwidth of ±16 kHz (128 pixels $\times$ 130 Hz/pixel).

Chemical shift artifact can be reduced to the degree that it is no longer apparent by using a high bandwidth. The downside is that high bandwidth images have a lower signal-to-noise ratio (SNR) (with the high bandwidth image appearing "grainy," as in both examples). Thus the choice of bandwidth is a compromise between the chemical shift that can be tolerated and SNR. The concept itself is also not that difficult to understand. When an individual echo (or signal) in MR is observed, typically 256 to 512 samples are taken (defining the resolution in the readout direction), with the Nyquist bandwidth being the reciprocal of the time between consecutive data samples. In most applications at 1.5 T, the bandwidth is chosen to be between 130 and 195 Hz/pixel. An alternative to using higher bandwidths, to avoid chemical shift artifact, is to employ fat saturation.

97 Geometric Distortion

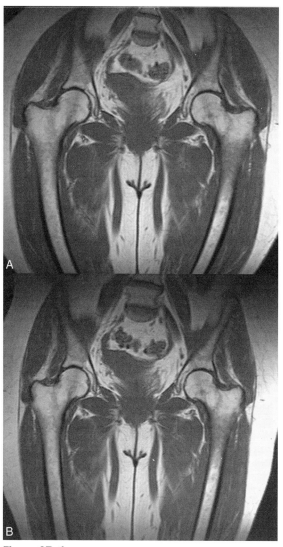

Figure 97–1

Fig. **97–1A,C** have substantial image distortion, especially at the periphery, secondary to nonlinear gradients. Virtually all MR systems suffer from gradient nonlinearity, often times due to coil design that seeks to optimize other gradient applications. It may be difficult on any one MR system to actually obtain an image depicting such spatial distortion, because postprocessing techniques, such as the use of a filter, may unknowingly be employed to correct the appearance of the image (Fig. **97–1B,D**).

Geometric distortion occurs commonly in MR. All forms of spatial distortion have to do with mismapping of signal data due to errors in phase or frequency. Small voxels will decrease the representation of distortion on the final image (although this does not change the actual distortion that occurs).

Distortion is due to a variety of factors, some intrinsic, others extrinsic to the subject being studied. During production of a magnet, despite attempts to create uniformity over the entire magnetic field, small inhomogeneities inevitably occur. In addition, gradient nonlinearity, in which along a given axis the magnetic field does not increase in a linear fashion, may exist due to gradient coil design. Such predictable factors that induce inhomogeneity and thus distortion can be corrected for. In the former instance, additional gradients, called shim gradients, may be used, which actually correct the distortion itself. In the latter instance, postprocessing methods correct the distortion

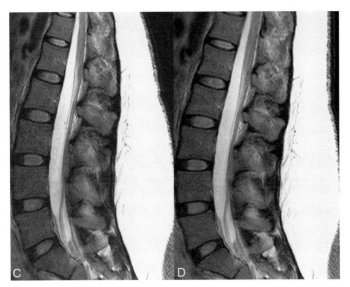

Figure 97–1 (Continued)

by remapping the incorrect spatial position so that it more accurately reflects the actual spatial position. Of importance, however, is that despite being able to correct for errors in spatial positioning, this technique cannot correct for the loss of spatial resolution that occurred due to the initial error in spatial encoding in regions of nonlinearity.

Unpredictable factors that cause distortion are inherently difficult to correct for. There are many such factors, including (1) internal distortions from chemical shift (see case 96) and differences in magnetic susceptibilities between tissues (see cases 93–94), both of which vary greatly from patient to patient; (2) moving objects and metal objects in and around the patient (see case 95); (3) eddy currents, currents created by rapidly turning on and off the gradients; and (4) incorrect gradient adjustments and calibrations. The latter is sometimes not corrected for simply because radiologists are unaware of such problems.

Geometric distortion is a significant issue that all radiologists should be aware of as it potentially can alter the interpretation of an exam. For example, in an image with spatial distortion, a specified axial slice in fact will be a curved plane (even if postprocessing methods make the final image appear without distortion). Thus, there can be a distinct mismatch between a specified slice and what the MR machine offers as being that slice. This could result in missing a small lesion that actually occurs in a slice other than the one designated. Realization of this common phenomenon is extremely important.

98 Motion: Ghosting and Smearing

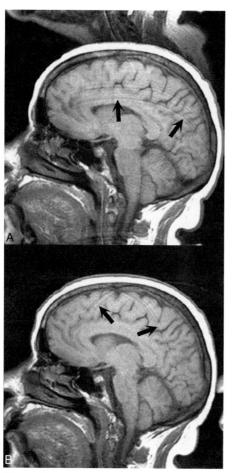

Figure 98–1

Ghosting typically occurs in the phase encoding direction, which is along the vertical axis in Fig. **98–1A** and the horizontal axis in Fig. **98–1B**. Note that wraparound artifact (see case 102) is present in both images also along the respective phase encoding axes. Fig. **98–1** and **98–2** display ghosts (arrows) caused by motion during acquisition of data that encodes edge information (high spatial frequency at the periphery of k space). Thus, motion artifact appears as edge-related ghosts of structures of high signal intensity. Fig. **98–2A** presents a T1-weighted axial image of the brain without motion artifact. With a small amount of motion (Fig. **98–2B**), a few ghosts appear, but with more substantial motion (Fig. **98–2C**), increased number and more defined ghosts appear. Discrete ghosts of the entire spatial information (not pictured) are caused by cyclic alteration in the MR signal from motion occurring throughout the period of data acquisition, often seen in pulsatile artifact (see case 101). Blurring (not pictured), another form of ghosting, is the loss of boundary definition due to slow modulation of the signal throughout data acquisition. Smearing (not pictured) occurs when signal is acutely disturbed during acquisition of the center lines of k space. It appears as smudging across a major portion of an axis (usually the phase encoding axis) from any structure that produces signal, not just those at the edges of the image.

Ghosting or ghost artifacts are mismapped signals of a part or all of a structure within a given image. The appearance of ghosts depends further on when and how alteration of signal occurs during data acquisition. Structures with high signal intensity (e.g., fat on a T1-weighted scan) have the highest propensity to cause ghosting. Although ghosting theoretically may occur in either the frequency encoding (readout) or phase encoding direction, it almost always occurs in the phase encoding direction. Data in the phase encoding direction takes a relatively long time to obtain (hundreds of milliseconds to minutes), and thus motion has ample opportunity to alter the MR

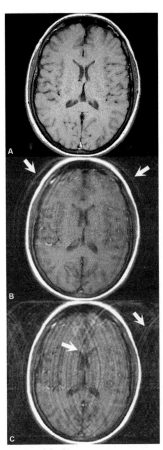

Figure 98–2

signal and cause artifact. This is in contradistinction to data acquisition in the frequency encoding direction, which takes only several milliseconds to occur. In such a short period of time, motion is not able to cause any significant artifact. Theoretically, if data acquisition in the frequency-encoding direction were to occur over a longer period of time, motion artifact might be seen in that direction. This, however, does not typically occur in clinical MR. Ghost artifacts may obscure true abnormalities or even mimic pathology. In addition, such artifact removes signal intensity from structures of interest (lowers the signal-to-noise ratio), and thus decreases one's ability to distinguish between adjacent tissues.

Improper encoding due to error induced by the MR unit or the environment causes ghosts. Motion either during or between sampling of echoes also causes ghosts. When motion occurs between MR echo sampling, data from a single point in the image may actually come from a different structure or different area within the same structure. Each view of the data point, therefore, will contain an MR signal with a different intensity. This results in a form of ghosting. Motion between sampling of echoes may be due to macroscopic physical motion. Macroscopic physical motion during a scan may be from patient movement, breathing, the cardiac cycle, bowel peristalsis, or pulsatile motion of large vessels (see case 101). Large pulsatile vessels may also cause artifact due to motion that occurs during echo sampling, leading to phase shifts and saturation effects.

99 Gradient Moment Nulling

Fig. **99–1A** and **99–1C** represent contrast-enhanced T1- and conventional T2-weighted images, respectively, with prominent motion artifacts (arrows) in the phase encoding direction. With the use of gradient moment nulling, artifact is markedly reduced and signal intensity is returned to dynamic structures of interest such as blood vessels (Fig. **99–1B**) and cerebrospinal fluid (CSF) (Fig. **99–1D**).

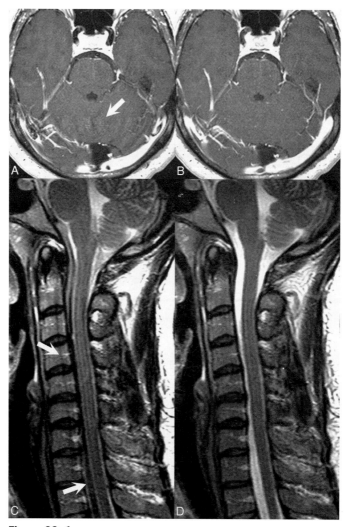

Figure 99–1

In scans of static objects, the rephasing gradient pulse successfully corrects for dephasing that occurs during the initial gradient pulse. With flow, however, the rephasing gradient pulse does not correct for added phase changes, resulting in dephasing and therefore artifact in the phase encoding direction (see case 101). The phase shifts that occur during the application of gradients relate to motion and gradient moments. Flow-related motion has three main dynamic components that contribute to artifact: constant velocity (first order), changing velocity or acceleration (second order), and changing acceleration, jerk, or pulsatility (third order). During the application of a gradient, each order of motion creates a phase component over the period of time the gradient is applied. Each phase component, termed a gradient moment, is referred to with respect to its associated order of motion (first-order motion is associated with first-order gradient moment, etc.). The total phase of a spin is then the sum of all the gradient moments.

Gradient moment nulling (GMN), also referred to as flow compensation, gradient moment rephasing (GMR), and motion artifact suppression technique (MAST), represents a common way to reduce errors caused by various orders of flow-related motion and the gradient moments created by such motion. This technique decreases the number of ghosts and returns signal intensity to the primary structure from which ghosting occurred. GMN involves the use of additional positive and negative gradients to null the net gradient moments of moving and stationary spins at the time data are collected. If stationary and moving spins have the same phase, signal will be correctly mapped. GMN may be used to correct for different orders of motion. In common clinical practice, correction for first-order motion is adequate for diagnostic purposes. This is due to the fact that the time between applications of gradient pulses during which phase shifts occur is so short that flow velocity is nearly constant within this period. For certain scan techniques, correction of higher order motion may be advantageous. However, the complexity and number of gradients applied increases for higher order motion.

Although motion is random in the x-, y-, and z-axes, GMN is effective when employed in the frequency encoding and slice selection directions. It is rarely utilized in the phase encoding direction because gradients in this direction are short and weak, and thus contribute little to overall phase shifts.

GMN does not increase the examination time. However, the lowest possible TE increases, especially for complex gradient pulsing. T1-weighted exams are especially sensitive to increases in TE as they rely on the use of a very short TE. This limits the ability of GMN to decrease flow artifact in T1-weighted scans. GMN is especially useful for T2-weighted scans and more so in the cervical and thoracic spine where CSF flow (pulsation) is greatest. Note that GMN increases the signal intensity of flowing fluids, which must be kept in mind when viewing the resultant images.

100 Spatial Saturation

Spatial saturation is an important technique for the reduction of motion artifacts, specifically ghosting (displaced false images of a body region). In this approach, an additional radiofrequency (RF) pulse is applied at the beginning of a pulse sequence to eliminate the signal from unwanted tissue. Magnetization in the area of the designated slab does not have sufficient time to recover (prior to the actual imaging part of the pulse sequence) and thus does not contribute to the observed signal.

A presaturation pulse can be applied either within (Fig. **100–1**) or parallel to (Fig. **100–2**) the imaging plane. The only difference between the two images in Fig. **100–1** is that a presaturation pulse (graphically shown by the label) has been applied during the acquisition of Fig. **100–1B**. This negates the signal from soft tissue anterior to the spine, preventing ghosting from motion therein propagating across the image. Note how much clearer the depiction is of the vertebral bodies and spinal cord with spatial saturation. For an in plane presaturation pulse to be effective, the direction of phase encoding must be such that the ghosts propagate and overlie the tissue of interest. Common applications include the spine (in sagittal or axial imaging if the phase encoding direction is anterior to posterior), the abdomen (to eliminate ghosting from the anterior abdominal wall), and the chest (to eliminate ghosting from the heart).

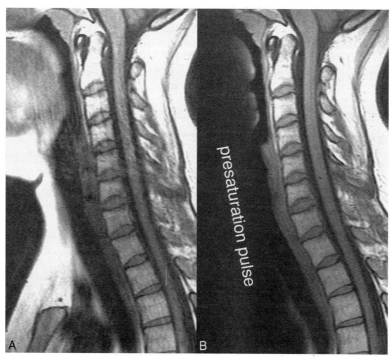

Figure 100–1

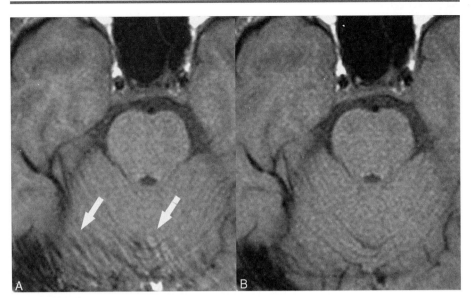

Figure 100–2

A less well appreciated application of spatial saturation is that illustrated in Fig. **100–2**, in which the presaturation pulse is applied parallel to the plane of imaging. Fig. **100–2A** is without, and Fig. **100–2B** is with presaturation. Note the pulsation artifacts (white arrows) from the transverse sinus that degrade visualization of the cerebellum in the image without the parallel presaturation pulse. In this comparison the depiction of the carotid arteries is also slightly improved. Blood that flows into a slice can have high signal intensity, with this phenomenon being the basis for time-of-flight MR angiography. Whether the flow is arterial or venous, this can produce substantial pulsation artifacts that degrade the image. By application of spatial saturation above and below the block of slices to be acquired, pulsation artifacts from arteries and veins can be markedly reduced. Common applications include imaging of the sella, internal auditory canals, and abdomen and pelvis (all for precontrast scans only).

The addition of a presaturation pulse, because it does require time to perform within the pulse sequence, may reduce the number of slices that can be acquired for a given TR. Another possible disadvantage is the additional heat deposition, if specific absorption rate (SAR) limits are a constraint.

101 Flow Artifacts

A T1-weighted axial gradient echo scan of the abdomen with fat saturation is illustrated in Fig. **101–1A**. Addition of spatial saturation pulses (see case 100), above and below the level of the slice, leads to loss of flow-related enhancement within the major veins (Fig. **101–1B**), which otherwise are high signal intensity. Prominent ghosts are noted from both the inferior vena cava and aorta along the phase encoding (vertical) axis on an axial T1-weighted fast spin echo (FSE) image (Fig. **101–1C**). Placement of a saturation pulse above the slice eliminates the ghosts from the aorta, but not the cava (arrows, Fig. **101–1D**), whereas a saturation pulse placed below the slice eliminates the ghosts from the cava but not the aorta (arrows, Fig. **101–1E**). Using

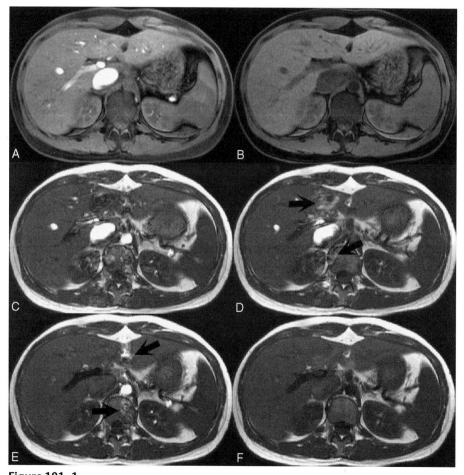

Figure 101–1

saturation pulses both above and below the slice largely eliminates these vascular ghosts (Fig. **101–1F**). Saturation pulses eliminate phase dispersion incurred by protons due to various flow-related phenomena (see below) essentially by demagnetizing all protons (causing loss of signal) prior to entry into a slice.

Flow may cause ghosting via multiple mechanisms, including phase shifts, time of flight (TOF), and saturation effects. In large vessels with rapid flow, macroscopic motion due to physiologic pulsation may also contribute to ghost artifacts (see case 98). Ghosts may be bright or dark depending on their phase relative to the background in which they occur. In pulsatile flow, the distance between such ghosts is dependent on the difference between TR and RR (the time between heartbeats). If TR and RR are completely in sync, ghosting will not occur.

As previously discussed, rephasing gradients correct for dephasing that occurs from initial gradients applied in the frequency encoding and section-selection axes. In a static object, all protons will then resonate coherently again. However, in flow, movement of protons from both Brownian motion and flow itself occurs between and during the dephasing and rephasing lobes of the gradient. This creates additional, unanticipated changes in phase (phase shifts), which translates into phase encoding errors that may result in ghosting.

Time of flight (see cases 41 and 42) and saturation effects may also contribute to flow artifact. With slow flow, protons present during the initial radiofrequency (RF) pulse are partially saturated and thus have lower signal intensity. However, protons entering an already excited slice are unsaturated (fully magnetized) and have high signal intensity. This phenomenon is called inflow enhancement and can be seen in both spin echo and gradient echo scans. With fast flow, in spin echo imaging, protons are exposed only to a 90° excitation pulse, but not the 180° refocusing pulse, resulting in low signal intensity. In gradient echo scans, as in 2D TOF angiography, fast flow may exaggerate inflow enhancement due to entry of unsaturated protons after the excitation pulse. The signal intensity of flow may thus be high or low depending on the scan technique and flow velocity (see case 40). In reality, flow does not strictly adhere to slow or fast phenomena or to an expected signal intensity. In fact, the signal intensity of flowing blood (or more generally any fluid, such as cerebrospinal fluid) may even change from echo to echo due to the mechanisms explained above, especially given the variable rate of flow in diastole and systole. During Fourier transformation, these differences cannot be logically accounted for and thus ghost artifacts result.

102 Aliasing

Fig. **102–1A,C,E** present various examples of aliasing, defined as wraparound of structures outside a specified field of view (FOV) to the opposite side of the image. The phase encoding direction is along the vertical axis in Fig. **102–1A** and **102–1E**, but along the horizontal axis in Fig. **102–1C**. In Fig. **102–1A** the neck is aliased to the top of the image (arrow). In Fig. **102–1C** the nose is wrapped around to the back of the head (arrow). In Fig. **102–1E** the top of the spine is aliased to the bottom of the image and vice versa. Increasing the FOV by oversampling eliminates aliasing (Fig. **102–1B,D,F**).

Aliasing can occur along any axis, including the frequency encoding, phase encoding, and in 3D imaging, along the slice selection axis. In the frequency encoding axis, sampling of an echo occurs at a rate known as the sampling bandwidth. The range of frequencies sampled increases with higher sampling bandwidths. However, the highest frequency that can be sampled unambiguously is a value termed the Nyquist frequency. Frequencies higher than the Nyquist frequency, which occur outside a specified FOV, falsely appear to originate from a lower frequency. This is because the incorrect frequency is the result of the actual frequency subtracted from the Nyquist frequency. The falsified frequency, then, acquires an opposite sign than it originally had and thus data wraps around to the opposite side of the frequency-encoding axis. With many modern MR systems, however, aliasing along the frequency encoding axis has been largely eliminated by automatic oversampling methods. Oversampling involves increasing the FOV, and thus increasing the number of sampled frequencies. This is typically done by increasing the sampling rate, without any change in overall acquisition time.

In the phase encoding axis, aliasing may also occur due to the same principles as noted above for the frequency encoding direction (i.e., the signal is not sampled "finely" enough to logically represent the signal distribution in the raw data). As with the frequency encoding axis, oversampling can eliminate wraparound. Oversampling in the phase encoding axis has the disadvantage of increasing scan time by a factor equal to the percent of oversampling (with all other factors held constant). However, it has the advantage of increasing the signal-to-noise ratio (see case 74).

In 3D imaging, aliasing may also occur in the slice selection axis if the slab excitation includes structures beyond what is phase encoded. Again, oversampling by increasing the number of phase encoding steps so that all of an excited slab is encoded can remove aliasing. Use of saturation pulses and removing extraneous slices from each end of an excitation slab are alternate methods of removing wraparound artifact.

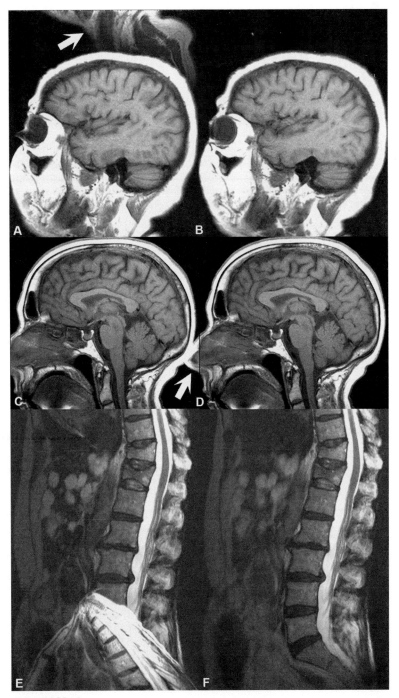

Figure 102–1

103 Truncation Artifacts

Fig. **103–1A** suffers from prominent truncation artifacts (black arrows) in the form of ringing (or "ring-down"), seen as alternating light and dark bands within the periphery of the brain. Fig. **103–2A** illustrates a syrinx-like artifact (white arrows) within the center of the thoracic cord on a T1-weighted sagittal scan, a classic truncation artifact that appears as a result of alternating dark and light signal bands overlying the spinal cord. This artifact is easily mistaken for hydromyelia (dilatation of the central canal, more commonly but incorrectly referred to as a "syrinx"), with the scan obtained in this instance in a normal, healthy volunteer. The artifacts in both scans result from an inappropriate choice of pixel size (too large). Truncation artifacts are reduced by the use of a smaller field of view (FOV) or a larger matrix size, the latter approach illustrated in both Figs. **103–1B** and **103–2B**.

The data acquired in k space (see case 10) for an MR image represents a finite amount of digital information due to the fact that the MR signal is sampled over a limited period of time. This inevitably leaves out (truncates) waveforms of data. Fourier transform (FT) analysis, the process by which MR data in k space is transformed into image pixel data via summation of sine and cosine waveforms, occurs then on a truncated amount of data. This results in deviation from the ideal signal intensity for any given image pixel. This phenomenon causes artifacts in particular in areas where signal changes abruptly, because FT analysis poorly accounts for such changes (it is better suited for gradual changes in signal intensity).

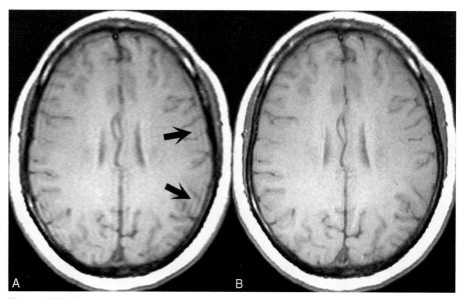

Figure 103–1

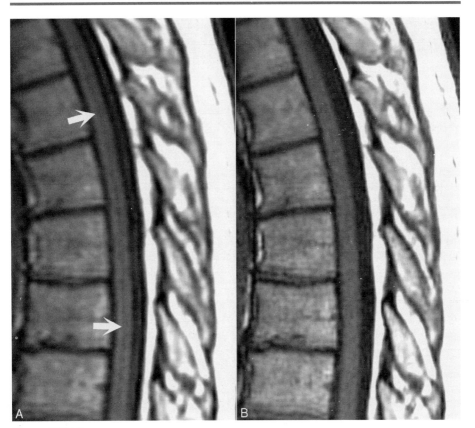

Figure 103–2

Truncation artifact, also referred to as "Gibbs' ringing" or edge-ringing artifact may appear in many ways: (1) "ringing," which involves alternating light and dark bands; (2) edge enhancement between areas of low and high signal intensity; (3) blurring between areas of low and high signal intensity; and (4) distortion of the size and shape of structures. Truncation artifacts can be diminished by several mechanisms. Decreasing the size of image pixels relative to the geometrical structures in the image, achieved by decreasing the FOV or increasing the matrix size, reduces the representation of the artifact on the final image. However, increasing the matrix size increases scan time and decreases the signal-to-noise ratio. Alternatively, decreasing the FOV may cause aliasing. These detrimental effects on image quality must be weighed against the possible benefit from removing the truncation artifact. Use of a filter that discards artifactual frequencies is another means of decreasing truncation artifact.

Index